M000307852

MEDICAL PRACTICE MANAGEMENT

Body of Knowledge Review
Second Edition

VOLUME 8

Risk Management

Medical Group Management Association
102 Inverness Terrace East
Englewood, CO 80112-5306
877.275.6462
mgma.com

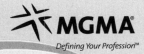

Defining Your Profession™

Medical Group Management Association® (MGMA®) publications are intended to provide current and accurate information and are designed to assist readers in becoming more familiar with the subject matter covered. Such publications are distributed with the understanding that MGMA does not render any legal, accounting, or other professional advice that may be construed as specifically applicable to an individual situation. No representations or warranties are made concerning the application of legal or other principles discussed by the authors to any specific factual situation, nor is any prediction made concerning how any particular judge, government official, or other person will interpret or apply such principles. Specific factual situations should be discussed with professional advisors.

PRODUCTION CREDITS
Publisher: Marilee E. Aust
Composition: Glacier Publishing Services, Inc.
Cover Design: Ian Serff, Serff Creative Group, Inc.

LIBRARY OF CONGRESS CATALOGING-IN-PUBLICATION DATA

Risk management.
    p. ; cm. — (Medical practice management body of knowledge review
(2nd ed.) ; v. 8)
   Includes bibliographical references and index.
   ISBN 978-1-56829-337-0
1. Medical offices—Risk management. I. Medical Group Management Association.
II. Series.
   [DNLM: 1. Practice Management—organization & administration. 2. Risk
Management—methods. W 80 R595 2008]
   R728.R497 2008
   610.68—dc22

                                                                2008044480

Copyright © 2009 Medical Group Management Association

All rights reserved. No part of this publication may be reproduced, stored in a retrieval system or transmitted, in any form or by any means, electronic, mechanical, photocopying, recording or otherwise, without the prior written permission of the copyright owner.

Printed in the United States of America
10 9 8 7 6 5 4 3 2 1

Dedication

To our colleagues in the profession
of medical practice management
and to the groups that support us
in our efforts to serve our profession.

Body of Knowledge Review Series — Second Edition

Contents

Preface

DESPITE VIEWPOINTS TO THE CONTRARY, risk management is not a function but a process.[1] It is a key process for business and is essential to protect the assets of the health care organization. These assets are not just the direct financial assets that could be endangered by a lawsuit, but they are also the intangible assets of lost opportunity, loss or diminished capability of personnel, loss or diminished usability of property, and the ever elusive loss of reputation and community trust.

Historically, risk management in health care has focused on losses incurred through medical malpractice.[2] Although certainly seen in most large, obvious losses, medical malpractice is only one component of the risk management process. In recent years, the focus has moved from clinical risk management, concentrated on losses directly related to clinical care, to a broader perspective. This perspective, known as enterprise risk management, considers all aspects of the organization's function as integrated components of overall loss exposure. Furthermore, in this framework, "risk" is synonymous with "capital." Risk exposure is therefore a direct potential loss of capital. Capital losses can come from operational exposures, financial risks, human capital risks, strategic risks, legal exposures, and technological risks.[3] In this risk management framework, the notion of risk management as a process tool rather than a "function" is not only reasonable, it is obvious.

Given that risk management cannot be relegated to a set of specific pieces of information but must be examined by parts of the process, this volume first examines the risk management process and then addresses the skills and tasks related to its effective execution.

Body of Knowledge Review Series Contributors

Geraldine Amori, PhD, ARM, CPHRM
Douglas G. Anderson, FACMPE
James A. Barnes, MBA
Fred Beck, JD
Jerry D. Callahan Jr., CPA
Anthony J. DiPiazza, CPA
David N. Gans, MSHA, FACMPE
Robert L. Garrie, MPA, RHIA
Edward Gulko, MBA, FACMPE, FACHE, LNHA
Kenneth T. Hertz, CMPE
Steven M. Hudson, CFP, CFS, CRPC
Jerry Lagle, MBA, CPA, FACMPE
Michael Landers
Gary Lewins, FACMPE, CPA, FHFMA
Ken Mace, MA, CMPE
Jeffrey Milburn, MBA, CMPE
Michael A. O'Connell, MHA, FACMPE, CHE
Dawn M. Oetjen, PhD, MHA
Reid M. Oetjen, PhD, MSHSA
Pamela E. Paustian, MSM, RHIA
David Peterson, MBA, FACMPE
Lisa H. Schneck, MSJ
Frederic R. Simmons Jr., CPA
Thomas E. Sisson, CPA
Donna J. Slovensky, PhD, RHIA, FAHIMA
Jerry M. Trimm, PhD, FHIMSS
Stephen L. Wagner, PhD, FACMPE
Lee Ann H. Webster, MA, CPA, FACMPE
Susan Wendling-Aloi, MPA, FACMPE
Warren C. White Jr., FACMPE
Lawrence Wolper, MBA, FACMPE, CMC
Lorraine C. Woods, FACMPE
James R. Wurts, FACMPE

Learning Objectives

AFTER READING THIS VOLUME, the medical practice executive will be able to accomplish the following tasks:

- Develop and implement a risk management plan to ensure a safe environment for patients, staff, and visitors;

- Develop and implement policies and procedures to manage the impact of adverse legal events;

- Establish a plan for disaster response and recovery; and

- Develop and implement a compliance program for federal and state laws and regulations.

Vignette **OSHA Inspection Nightmares**

◢ Tales of Recent OSHA Inspections

A small medical practice in Michigan – ABC Clinic* – sustained hefty fines when a disgruntled employee complained to the Occupational Safety and Health Administration (OSHA) that her employer had not switched to safety needles. Although OSHA found the practice was out of compliance in several areas, the staff's handling of the inspection actually racked up the fines. Why? When an OSHA inspector arrived unannounced at ABC Clinic, he was greeted warmly by the receptionist. After showing his credentials, he asked to be escorted to the clinical area. The staff allowed him to wander freely around the practice! Three hours later, the inspector left with a briefcase full of citations amounting to several thousand dollars. The physicians and staff were shocked two weeks later when they received a 15-page list of penalties. The group wrote a check to OSHA that week.

In another case initially related to safety needles, a practice employee at ABC Group in California who had been accidentally pricked with a contaminated needle called the local OSHA office and lodged a formal complaint against her employer, which had previously refused to offer safety needles to employees. OSHA soon visited the office and discovered more than $40,000 worth of violations. The employer negotiated to get the fines reduced by $20,000.

*Names have been changed to protect the identity of the practice.

In a different type of case, a disgruntled employee in Idaho called OSHA, reporting that his employer, ABC Family Practice, didn't have an OSHA manual and that patient areas weren't disinfected often enough. The surprised administrator received a three-page letter from OSHA containing the employee's allegations and demanding a written response and copies of all applicable OSHA policies.

OSHA has inspected thousands of physicians' offices in the last few years. The most common citations were for violations of the Bloodborne Pathogens Standard and the Hazard Communication Standard.

What would happen if an OSHA inspector visited your medical practice today? Practice administrators must continually assess their offices' potential risks to prevent malpractice suits, loss control issues, and government claims of abuse and noncompliance. Risk management is an integral part of mastering the art of the medical practice executive's job.

Current Risk Management Issues

◢ The Risk Management Process

To fully appreciate the ramifications and breadth of issues involved in risk management, it is essential to understand the risk management process.

Risk management as a process has four essential components:

1. *Risk assessment and analysis* – identification and analysis of exposures;

2. *Loss control* – identification and selection of potential mechanisms for addressing those exposures;

3. *Risk financing* – using selected techniques including risk financing, for failed control of losses; and

4. *Monitoring* – continuous monitoring of selected methods for controlling losses for potential improvement.[4]

These components applied to financial, human, operational, property, technological, and strategic areas across all aspects of the organization create the constellation that defines the organization's risk management program. What this means for the medical practice executive is related to the executive's ability to assess risks.

■ Risk Assessment and Analysis

The medical practice executive must ensure that he or she is aware of all potential risk exposures. As James Reason discusses in his book *Human Error*, every process contains latent errors, many of which are identified as such because our systems rely on consistently perfect human activity.[5] In fact, many processes depend on human vigilance and omniscient foresight to stop errors from occurring. Examples on a grand scale include the lack of coordination of resources early in the 9/11 tragedy and, more recently, the disorder that resulted in the loss of lives and chaos after Hurricane Katrina.[6]

On a smaller, but still significant scale are those preventable failures that result in medication errors, fires on site, staff injury, failures of service initiatives, or loss of business productivity due to technology failures. In each of those circumstances, the blame often is laid on the person who "didn't follow the policy" or "didn't pay close enough attention." In fact, processes without risk control mechanisms to counter the human factor are fraught with latent errors. The opportunities for error can become aligned through serendipitous occurrences, or through a series of small human errors that can ultimately result in devastating outcomes and losses. Reason's "Swiss Cheese Model," often quoted in patient safety literature, is applicable to all aspects of an organization's processes and activities. The alignment of any number of process "holes" can result in risk management exposures. The key is to find where those latent exposures lie before losses occur. [7]

Ultimately, the most exhaustive way to identify potential exposures in complex systems is through a process, such as a failure modes and effects analysis (FMEA). This process, which gained popularity through its use in engineering, is designed to examine every step of a process and identify the myriad ways in which each step could fail, as well as the potential for that failure to be stopped.[8] Nevertheless, even a tool as powerful as FMEA is limited by resources. Such analyses take time. Obvious loss potential areas may justify the dedication of human capital for this type of intensive analysis. Nonetheless, many processes have the potential to lead to equally devastating losses. How then does an organization prioritize the processes to review?

Information on exposures that have high loss potential can be gathered from a number of sources. The organization's own insurance claims and malpractice loss runs are basic sources of information. Complaints from patients and/or staff are another fundamental source of information. Formal risk assessments by outside consultants, self-assessment questionnaires, literature reviews, and insurance application forms also provide exposure identification. Furthermore, by examining the questions on the insurance application or survey forms, the executive can ascertain which processes are perceived as high risk by insurers and other surveyors. Finally, by using a simple but effective technique, staff can list the various processes in each department and then ask "What can go wrong?" for each process. If answered honestly, it will be apparent from the list where loss control mechanisms might be useful.

Loss Control

The next step in the risk management process is to analyze the data and identify the tools that will reduce either the frequency (loss prevention)[9] or the severity (loss reduction)[10] of losses. The potential losses prime for application of these techniques are (1) those that occur frequently even though the cost per loss may be small (e.g., missed appointments or employee unplanned absences); and (2) those that occur infrequently but are more costly per loss (e.g., medical malpractice claims). Furthermore, as stated earlier, any process that relies heavily on human compliance with complex procedures (or procedures in a complex environment) is subject to great variability and potential error.

Those areas in any process in which high variability or high potential for loss exists should be addressed first. Potential methods to address these issues can be found in the industry literature or through insurance or business consultants. Nonetheless, a key point to remember is that loss control methods are not uniformly applicable in all situations. The unique location, culture, and characteristics of each organization may render a solution a potentially bad fit. Consequently, each considered solution must be analyzed for its potential latent failures in the given situation.

Planning and Preparedness for Catastrophic Events

Losses stemming from natural disasters provide examples of the variability needed in loss control methods. Flood and emergency evacuation processes that worked in Vermont in the ice storm of 2000 were not uniformly applicable to New Orleans in 2005 in the face of Hurricane Katrina. Both were water- and wind-based disasters. Both affected the availability of electricity and potable water. Both affected transportation. Both created temperature conditions that were dangerous to humans (the ice storm resulted in deaths by freezing and collision; the hurricane, in deaths by drowning and heat). Both required evacuation of vast numbers of people from nursing homes and hospitals. However, unlike the aftermath of Katrina, the New England ice storm did not result in potential infectious disease through coliform or mosquito transmission, and it did not result in the decay of human remains. In addition, the repair time and the time before people could return to their homes after the ice storm was shorter. Although there certainly is much to be learned from the communication among various agencies, the military, and first responders such as emergency service personnel, many other aspects of the emergency plan do not go far enough to meet the needs of a different type of water- and wind-based disaster.

In addition to natural and human-made disasters, increasing attention is being paid to the threat of an influenza pandemic. Medical practices should review disaster preparedness protocols and procedures in their organizations and in their communities to be up to date on the incorporation of pandemic influenza preparedness into emergency management procedures and what their own roles and responsibilities would be at that time.

The Department of Health and Human Services (HHS) and the Centers for Disease Control and Prevention (CDC) have published a number of resources specifically targeted to help medical offices and ambulatory clinics assess and improve their preparedness for responding to pandemic influenza. Medical practices may find that they need to adapt the information and checklists to meet their unique needs.

Given the rapidly changing nature of pandemic influenza information at the federal, state, and local levels, medical practices should monitor the Websites of the HHS (www.hhs.gov/pandemicflu) and CDC (www.cdc.gov/flu), as well as other selected Websites for new and updated information. The Website www.pandemicflu.gov contains links to state pandemic influenza emergency plans, which medical practice leadership and staff should review and use to complement their overall plan.

According to the CDC, medical offices should develop a structure for planning and decision making. The structure should include a planning committee with both clinical (physicians, nurses, and ancillary staff) and administrative (medical practice administrator and support staff) representation, as well as the services of an environmentalist, if possible. One person in the organization, such as the practice administrator, should be assigned responsibility for coordinating preparedness planning for the practice. A point of contact (either someone in the clinic or an outside consultant) should be responsible for answering questions and/or providing consultation on infection control to prevent transmission of pandemic influenza. The organizational structure should be described in a written pandemic influenza plan.

The plan developed for the practice should be consistent with existing practice emergency/disaster plans and with community response plans. The key elements of an influenza pandemic plan for prepared medical practices are:

- A plan for surveillance and detection of pandemic influenza in the population served;
- A communication plan;
- Provision for an education and training program to ensure that all personnel understand the implications of, and control measures for, pandemic influenza;
- Informational materials for patients on pandemic influenza, which are language and reading-level appropriate for the

population being served, including a means to distribute these materials[11];

- A plan for triage and management of patients during a pandemic;

- An infection control plan[12];

- A vaccine and antiviral use plan; and

- An occupational health plan that addresses issues related to surge capacity (i.e., dealing with an influx of patients as well as a shortage of staff and supplies) during a pandemic.[13]

In these extreme examples of actual and potential disasters, the same principle applies to any proposed loss control solution. No loss control mechanism should be selected without full consideration of the influence of local cultural and environmental conditions on the potential for failure. Even apparently fail-proof plans may fall short because of unforeseen events. The World Trade Center buildings were built to withstand potential encounters with airplanes. However, the World Trade Center was built many years before the Boeing 767s, which ultimately hit the towers, had even been designed.[14]

High Reliability Organizations

In the risk management selection process, consideration should be given to developing procedures that increase a system's reliability. This should include any mechanism that reduces variability through human fatigue or physical condition, variance in the physical environment, and reliance on human vigilance. The concept of the high reliability organization (HRO), originally studied at the University of California at Berkeley, is being applied throughout clinical care organizations to address the issue of providing care in complex systems under complex conditions.[15] Although based on industries for which safety is a key issue, such as aviation or nuclear energy, high-reliability concepts also apply to health care processes, where error can also result in significant loss.[16]

HROs have certain characteristics that contribute to consistent outcomes. Among the most salient are their flexibility when it comes to decision making and organization. Whoever has the information or appropriate skill can assume responsibility as the situation dictates. Bureaucracy is adaptable to the needs at hand. Furthermore, HROs are obsessed with reliability to the point of trumping efficiency. Their culture communicates and supports the value of reliability, and it rewards people for exhibiting the desired behavior in critical situations. Finally, organization employees are taught to maintain awareness of the situation and to make efforts to understand situations that do not seem right, rather than to ignore them or to assume that it is the job of someone higher on the administrative level, and they are reinforced in these efforts.

Along with these traits are tools that are designed to reduce variability in action by reducing reliance on vigilance, memory, or habit. Those tools include checklists, clearly defined procedures that are supported by reminders and lists, task simplification to reduce the number of steps, a reduction in the number of hand-offs, and automatic correction on critical steps.[17] It is impossible to predict everything, however. Given that, it is essential that appropriate risk financing be available to cover unforeseen losses.

Risk Financing

Most executives are familiar with the risk-financing vehicles of commercial insurance and self-insured vehicles, such as captives, risk retention groups, and trusts. What many executives may not fully appreciate, though, is that commercial insurance, although more costly, is effectively a contractual transfer of risk.[18] The risk of loss belongs to the insurer. Consequently, the risk of financial devastation through catastrophic events is minimized for the organization. The downside to risk transfer is that the insurance company maintains control over what will be covered and retains the ability to increase premiums. Furthermore, the premium paid by the organization is not based solely on the organization's history nor specifically on its loss control efforts but on an aggregate of similar organizations with combined loss experience. Of course, some attention is paid to the organization's specific loss history; however, the cost of overhead and need for margin to the insurance company sometimes outweigh those benefits.

Risk transfer is not bad. For forms of losses that are unpredictable and potentially costly (e.g., automobile, directors' and officers' liability, employment liability, property, key person), commercial insurance is the standard and probably most cost-effective form of risk financing. The organization hopes to never need it. Nonetheless, it would be extremely difficult to predict ultimate losses and to plan for setting aside sufficient funds to cover these losses should they occur.

Self-insurance vehicles are best when there is a known frequency and consistent value of typical losses.[19] The organization must have sufficient funds set aside to cover those losses. Self-insurance vehicles tend to be less expensive to administer and offer the organization more control over the loss control mechanisms and their effect on the premium.

In addition, there are losses that occur infrequently but result in such large losses that it is better to cover them with more structured forms of risk financing. For minimal losses or extremely infrequent losses, risk financing might include loans, nonfunded reserves, or even payment from the operations budget.

Given the variety of options for risk financing, it is essential that the medical practice executive understand the full array of potential risks faced by the organization and plan accordingly for failure in any arena. Does the organization have a plan to respond to a disaster that affects all technological equipment? Is there a plan should delivery of medical supplies be cut off? Is there a plan for a loss of water or electricity, for a contagious illness reducing the availability of staff to care for patients, or for severe weather resulting in patients and staff being forced to remain in the building for days? What is the plan should an intruder hold staff hostage? The number of risks that must be provided for and covered both through procedures and possible risk-financing mechanisms is seemingly unlimited.

◼ Monitoring

Time changes all things. The methods and procedures that work at one time can suddenly no longer fit the organization's practice. The challenge is to remain attuned to the influence of organizational change on loss control methods. Once a method of loss control is chosen, the tendency is to be so desirous of it working that signs that it is not working are ignored. Monitoring and reevaluation of all loss control methods, therefore, must occur regularly.

Standardized times should be scheduled for review of written policies and procedures as well as actual processes as performed in the organization. A standard timetable for review will ensure that the organization is regularly updating all aspects of its risk management program.

Knowledge Needs

ACCORDING TO the American College of Medical Practice Executives, there are four key skills, or knowledge needs, required of the medical practice executive for effective execution of the risk management process. Those skills can be grouped in alignment with the steps of the process described in the previous section.

Risk Assessment and Analysis Skills

1. Continually assess potential medical practice risks to help avert malpractice suits, address loss control issues, and deter government claims of abuse.

2. Interpret government regulations on corporate compliance and fraud/abuse issues and inform physicians and staff to promote adherence.

3. Negotiate contracts (including capitation agreements) with payers, contractors, vendors, and other outside resources to eliminate risks for the practice.

Loss Control Skills

4. Communicate consistently to medical practice staff via the most appropriate media the commitment to minimizing risk and maximizing compliance to ensure high-quality patient care.

5. Build and maintain a relationship with legal counsel to ensure the most appropriate resources on practice liability matters.

6. Plan security systems and training to minimize possible workplace violence in the medical facility.

7. Write and communicate clear policies on medical practice risk and compliance matters, including medical records, self-referrals, and patient safety, to limit risk exposure.

8. Investigate all claims against the practice, its physicians, and staff to ensure that all parties are treated fairly and correctly.

Risk-Financing Skills

9. Report regularly to the board, administrators, and staff on risk-related matters to ensure up-to-date understanding of liability issues for the practice.

Monitoring Skills

10. Evaluate future risks for the practice in light of past history, present conditions, and forecasted trends to ensure adequate preparation for the future.[20]

Clearly, there is overlap and redundancy in the risk management process. Monitoring skills are also assessment skills. Risk-financing skills are part of monitoring skills as well as risk-reduction techniques. It is not reasonable to expect the medical practice executive to possess all of the skills required of a risk manager. However, it is reasonable to expect the executive to recognize any discrepancy between his or her personal skill set and the required skills for the job and to seek the services of a professional risk manager if needed. Most important, the medical practice executive should have a firm grasp of all loss exposures faced by the organization and be able to recognize when the resources for addressing those exposures may have to be sought from outside the organization.

Chapter 1   # Ensuring a Safe Environment for Patients, Staff, and Visitors

◢ Managing Staff Safety[21]

One of the most important interpersonal relationships within the group practice is the one between the employee and the supervisor. Management reflects its culture through the supervisors' attitudes towards employees in the workplace. Therefore, healthy relationships are critical to the success of the group practice. The group practice should strive to provide a healthy work environment, encourage employees to perform at their best, and become known in the community as a great place to work.

Management decisions affect the cost of delivery of health care services, which ultimately affects consumers. The whole purpose of employee relations is to attract, develop, and retain high performers. This section addresses key issues regarding the critical aspects of employee relations to improve working conditions, provide a safe environment, and increase productivity. The section ends with a discussion of labor organization and representation focusing on the unionization of health care professionals.

Introduction to Employee Safety, Health, and Security

Employers realize how important occupational health and safety programs are to maintaining a productive and highly efficient workforce. The cost of unsafe and unhealthy conditions in the workplace is substantial considering the lost productivity due to accidents and illness. In addition, the cost of health care benefits to the employer continues to rise, contributing to higher health insurance costs when employees are injured. The cost of providing safety and training programs is low when compared to the cost of employee accidents, injuries and illnesses, and workers' compensation claims.

More important than the economic aspect of health and safety is the employee's right to work in an environment that does not pose a health hazard or an unreasonable risk of injury. No employer wishes to see anyone harmed by the group's everyday operations, but failure to establish and enforce strict health and safety policies may unintentionally encourage careless practices.

Today, the rise of worldwide disasters and the possible risks to health care workers and patients make such policies even more critical. For example, pregnant employees or those attempting to become pregnant should not provide care to patients with a known diagnosis of cytomegalovirus, acquired immunodeficiency syndrome, ARC, or human immunodeficiency virus. Issues related to significant exposure to blood, body fluids, and tissues must be addressed, as well as exposure to contaminated needles, instrument punctures, and lacerations. Another growing concern is exposure to Hepatitis B and the need to administer the Hepatitis B vaccine to those employees involved with direct patient care and supply handling.

Finally, employers have become aware of the importance of protecting the environment, community, and society in which they work. Employers realize that they are a part of the community and must take a role in protecting and enhancing that community. A record of occupational health and safety problems is a detriment to the employer's image and place within the community.

Employee Safety

The Occupational Safety and Health Act of 1970

A major federal law affecting employers is the Occupational Safety and Health Act of 1970. The law was passed in part to solve some of the inadequacies that were thought to exist in state workers' compensation laws. The law encourages employers and employees to work toward reducing the number of hazards in the workplace. It also stimulates employers and employees to develop new programs, or revise existing ones, to provide safe and healthful working conditions.

The act requires that every employer covered by the law provide employees with a place of employment that is free from recognized hazards to life or health. The act further provides that each employee comply with all standards, rules, regulations, and orders issued by the employers to comply with the law. An employer covered by the act is defined as any person who has employees and who is engaged in interstate commerce. The act provides for civil and criminal penalties for violation of the law or regulations issued thereunder.

OSHA Tuberculosis Enforcement Guidelines

On May 7, 1992, the Occupational Safety and Health Administration (OSHA) issued its "OSHA Enforcement Guidelines for Occupational Exposure to Tuberculosis." The guidelines covered employee training, skin testing, isolation procedures, patient transport requirements, and record-keeping. The guidelines also proposed standards for respirator use in contaminated areas. The guidelines were effective only in New York, New Jersey, Puerto Rico, and the Virgin Islands. However, OSHA considered issuing national standards for the control of TB contamination.

On September 14, 1992, the National Institute for Occupational Safety and Health (NIOSH) issued its own "Recommended Guidelines for Personal Respiratory Protection of Workers in Healthcare Facilities Potentially Exposed to Tuberculosis." The NIOSH standard requires use on high-efficiency particulate filters in suspected contaminated areas.

Finally, on October 18, 1994, the national Centers for Disease Control and Prevention issued final guidelines for preventing TB transmission. The final guidelines recommend that a health care provider implement and enforce a TB infection control plan program. The guidelines also suggest the use of personal respiratory protective equipment in areas of potential TB exposure. As a result, medical practices should have a tuberculin skin test policy and appropriate follow-up.

OSHA Bloodborne Pathogen Standard

On December 2, 1991, OSHA issued its "Occupational Exposure to Bloodborne Pathogens Standards." This regulation requires employees to identify tasks and procedures and job classifications where occupational exposure to blood or other bodily fluid occurs and requires "universal precautions" to be taken in regard to treatment of all bodily fluids. The standard requires employers to require, provide, and replace personal protective equipment and to provide postexposure follow-up evaluations for any exposure incident at no cost to employees.

Numerous state and local regulations also affect health and safety in the workplace. The medical group should be aware of these laws and conform to them.

Why Is an Employee Safety and Health Policy So Important?

The physical condition of the workplace generally has an effect on employees' productivity, attitude, and organizational morale. For these reasons, most employers take aggressive steps to provide a pleasant, clean, and safe work environment. If working conditions are not pristine, employees may suffer from lost time on the job because of occupational accidents and injuries. Therefore, personal health and safety have become increasingly important to employers. Workers' compensation claims continue to increase and demand close oversight by management.

Safe work practices that are followed and enforced help to ensure not only that workers are kept out of danger, but also that risk of damage to the group practice's property and liability status is minimal. Thus, employers must establish policies to guide managers, supervisors, and employees in obeying safety and health regulations.

For customizable policies on Exposure Control and Hazard Communication, please refer to the Medical Group Management Association *Operating Policies & Procedures Manual for Medical Practices*, third edition.

Why Is Delegating Safety Responsibilities to an Individual Important?

Most small medical groups choose to select an individual to be responsible for safety in the workplace. Larger medical practices may appoint a safety officer for this role. Management should develop a comprehensive safety program suited to the group's particular needs.

Because much of safety and health compliance lies in providing educational safety and health training programs, sometimes these safety functions are combined with training. Another option is to establish a safety committee responsible for all safety and health programs. Safety incentive programs are another way to ensure compliance with regulations. Employees who do not follow the safety policies should be properly disciplined to ensure that safety regulations are followed.

Finally, safety has become an overriding concern in health care institutions because they may have patients who are incapable of helping themselves in emergencies. Fire is one of the most dangerous emergencies. Therefore, a fire plan should be included in the policy manual, and fire safety training should be provided for all employees. Other areas to consider in the safety policy are:

- On-the-job injuries;
- Accident and injury reports;
- Medical emergencies;
- Posting of emergency information;
- Evacuation plan;
- First aid equipment;

- Weather-related alerts;
- Care and use of equipment;
- Terrorism threats;
- Bomb threats;
- Protective clothing;
- Safety inspections;
- Reporting of unsafe conditions;
- Firearms;
- Safety designated areas;
- Safety suggestions; and
- Incentive award programs.

Employee Security

Because of vandalism, pilferage, thefts, bomb scares, terrorism, and major incidences of workplace violence, most group practices realize that securing their facilities has become very important. For example, the theft of business equipment, especially small items, has greatly increased in recent years and is very costly to employers. Computer hacking and viruses have generated their own security precautions. As terrorism and workplace violence continue to affect the lives of employees and employers, security programs have become a top priority.

Security programs involve taking precautionary measures to ensure adequate protection of the group practice's property and assets, as well as that of its employees. Many health care managers have written and unwritten security rules that range from "the last one out locks up for the night" to contracting security firms for surveillance. A group practice's security needs vary depending on its location, the nature of its operations, and number of employees. Some larger groups hire security consultants to develop and administer their security programs.

A typical security program requires all employees to wear identification (ID) badges while at work, which helps prevent unauthorized entry and possible theft. Secured doors to authorized-only areas may involve coded or card locks. More sophisticated security techniques include motion sensors, video surveillance, spot inspections, fingerprint scans, retina scans, or security guards on site. Clearly visible ID badges help to quickly identify unauthorized people on medical group property and help prevent acts of terrorism.

Managers should take terrorism very seriously. The possibility of using everyday substances as biochemical weapons is a threat to both individuals and health care providers. Controlled substances should be kept in a secure place, and only authorized individuals should have access.

Workplace Violence

Workplace violence is a very real threat in our daily working lives. In 2003, workplace violence accounted for about 16 percent of on-the-job deaths, while the cost of injuries is incalculable. This percentage is a dramatic increase over the single-digit figure of the early 1980s. According to the Bureau of Labor Statistics, homicide is the second leading cause of job-related deaths for men and the single leading cause for women. The incident rate for workplace violence in the health care sector is 5.2. To compare the incident rate of one's group practice to this average, refer to the Bureau of Labor Statistics Website (www.bls.gov).

Most attackers and harassers are people the victims deal with on a daily basis. Co-workers and supervisors account for most of the harassers at work; customers, clients, and patients account for the largest group of attackers at work. Typical perpetrators of workplace violence are bitter, dissatisfied people who make threats of violence. Other types include:

- Frustrated employees who are shuffled from low-level tasks to even lower-level tasks;
- Frustrated professionals;
- Those who refuse to accept blame for their own problems;
- Those with pent-up rage;
- Those experiencing substance abuse;

- Those experiencing extreme stress in their personal lives or with their jobs; and

- Those with little or no support systems such as families or friends.

Characteristics of at-risk work environments include group practices with:

- A strict authoritarian management style;

- Numerous grievances filed;

- Many disciplinary actions and/or terminations;

- Inconsistent, inequitable, or insensitive management;

- Chronic labor-management disputes;

- Multiple injury claims;

- Frequent layoffs and downsizing;

- Disgruntled employees;

- Interpersonal conflicts on the job; and

- Failure to recognize and intervene early in the cycle of violence.

Although this list is not exhaustive, it does illustrate typical factors associated with workplace violence. Experts warn that in most cases where violence has occurred, there were indicators of potential or impending violence before it actually occurred. Ineffective or incompetent management contributes to workplace violence by:

- Not promptly responding to pre-employment warning signs or clues of future violence;

- Not admitting that a potentially violent situation has occurred;

- Not following up after warning behaviors;

- Not communicating an expectation of self-control to the involved employee; and

- Not communicating that the employee will be held responsible for his or her inappropriate and unacceptable behavior.

The emotional and psychological toll on employees subjected to workplace violence can be devastating. Three out of four workers who have experienced workplace violence report having suffered psychological and emotional distress. As a result, an employer's work effectiveness and productivity may be severely damaged. In addition to physical and emotional costs, workplace violence can have a dramatic impact on an employer's financial resources. Employers pay more than $4.2 billion each year because of workplace violence. The average cost of a single incident is $250,000. Workplace violence also affects workers' morale and productivity, increases absenteeism, promotes worker turnover, and raises costs for security and workers' compensation.

Who Is Held Responsible for Workplace Violence?

The work environment is critical to employee morale. People enjoy their work for a variety of reasons, but atmosphere is key to employee retention and the prevention of workplace violence. On the whole, average pay combined with excellent working conditions are much preferred to high pay coupled with horrible working conditions. Employees want to like their work, their peers, and their supervisors.

Federal and state occupational safety and health agencies have taken a more aggressive stance in enforcing an employer's statutory duty to provide employees with a working environment free of harm. Such agencies have found this duty to include an obligation to provide a working environment free from violence. In addition, state legislatures have begun to implement statutory mandates that ensure employers take precautions to minimize workplace violence.

A good way is to focus on encouraging trust by facilitating open communication. These prevention strategies should be considered:

- Training managers and supervisors to recognize early clues and warning signs of potential violence;
- Training workers in the techniques of conflict management and resolution;
- Striving to reduce or eliminate workplace stress;

- Recognizing and rewarding outstanding work and unique contributions;

- Establishing procedures for handling grievances – including listening and responding with empathy and sensitivity to employee concerns and grievances;

- Assisting employees in problem-solving, and referring employees to other resources when appropriate;

- Providing personal counseling for staff;

- Administering discipline consistently;

- Providing employees with written documentation and being clear about what behavior is expected to correct a problem;

- Administering termination, if warranted, with empathy and compassion, and backing it up with documentation;

- Implementing security programs that protect employees from internal and external risks; and

- Setting up a crisis plan.

What can be done to protect the workplace (and its financial resources) from violence? It can best be protected by developing and enforcing strong workplace safety policies and procedures for antici-pating, handling, and investigating potentially violent situations. Such policies and procedures should provide proper guidance and communication channels for supervisors and employees who may be exposed to violence in the workplace.

Appropriate workplace safety policies should include the following:

- Designating an interdisciplinary management task force that is responsible for creating, evaluating, and ensuring imple-mentation of the employer's workplace safety policies, con-ducting security and safety assessments, developing security plans, improving lighting in parking lots (the greatest areas of liability for workplace violence), and providing training for specially designated individuals to enforce security;

- Training supervisors and department heads to anticipate and analyze potential problems, recognize signs of potential conflict, and respond to potential volatile situations in ways that minimize their escalation;

- Educating employees about the potential danger of workplace violence and the proper response procedures for voicing concerns or complaints;

- Adding mechanical and electronic security devices to enhance employee protection;

- Creating procedures for investigating complaints of employee indiscretions and work incidents that indicate a potential for violence;

- Training designated people or contract professionals to provide emergency aid to victims of violence;

- Establishing procedures for pre-employment screening by conducting background checks and security evaluations of job applicants;

- Creating procedures for ensuring adequate training and supervision of employees; and

- Establishing procedures for alerting community law enforcement agencies when appropriate.

Supervisors and department heads should be specially trained to recognize the signs of potential violence. Management should be alerted to an employee who becomes romantically obsessed with a co-worker, visitor, or patient; engages in stalking or other harassing behavior; threatens or intimidates another employee with expressed or implied threats of violence; or engages in excessive discussion of weapons.

Workplace violence is rarely an isolated incident. Rather, workplace violence is a growing pattern of behaviors. An employee who exhibits paranoid or other outrageous behavior or exhibits extreme job-related or personal stress should raise concern. Any employee who brings a weapon to the workplace should be immediately reprimanded in accordance with the employer's disciplinary policies.

Employee investigations often become necessary when an employee has committed misconduct, exhibited poor work performance, engaged in violent or threatening behavior, or otherwise raised suspicions that they are unfit and possibly dangerous. The practice executive has a legal obligation to investigate all credible information indicating that the employee poses a potential threat of violence. This obligation might include conducting employee searches and using surveillance of electronic communications.

Conducting Employee Searches

Managerial guidelines should clearly define when, where, and how the practice may conduct searches of the employee's person or personal property. Employees should be notified that their person and personal property may be subjected to search by the employer at any time. The employer should retain the right to search all computers, including e-mail messages, lockers, offices, filing cabinets, and desks used by staff.

A "reasonable" search is one that balances the employee's expectation of privacy against the employer's legitimate business needs. The practice executive can lower an employee's "expectation of privacy" and take more discretion in conducting employee searches by simply informing employees that their person and property may be subject to search by the employer at any time.

Surveillance of Electronic Communications

Employees also have a reasonable expectation of privacy when engaging in telephone conversations and other electronic communications. State and federal privacy laws may impose liability on an employer for attempting to monitor such communications without the permission of the employee and other relevant parties. An employer should not attempt to monitor electronic communications without legal advice.

In developing and enforcing any workplace safety policy, a practice must balance workplace safety concerns against employee privacy rights. A practice may expose itself to liability from an accused employee for claims of defamation, wrongful discharge, invasion of privacy, fraud and misrepresentation, intentional and negligent infliction of emotional distress, breach of an implied employment contract or an implied covenant of good faith and fair dealing, assault, battery, false imprisonment, or discrimination in violation of equal opportunity and anti-discrimination laws. It is, therefore, very important for the group practice to consider its legal rights and obligations before implementing any workplace safety program.

The increasing acts of violence in the workplace should make us aware of violence and the vulnerabilities everyone may face as we enter our working environments. Having appropriate policies and procedures for limiting violence can enable the practice to control the workplace and limit exposure.

An excellent resource for learning more about workplace violence is the National Organization for Victim Assistance.

Monitoring Techniques

Risk exposure monitoring must happen on a regular and ongoing basis. It is essential that the medical practice executive understand the limitations and demands of both federal and state laws that apply to employees, premises liability, and visitors. Furthermore, to protect the organization, the medical practice executive should be conversant on state-permitted use of property surveillance, permissible drug testing of employees, and permitted use of pre-employment physicals and reference checks.

Recipients of federal funds are mandated to comply with the Drug-Free Workplace Act of 1988, which requires employers to have a drug-free awareness program and drug-free policies. Employees must be aware that drug use, manufacture, or distribution is not permitted in the workplace. Furthermore, any convictions related to drugs must be reported to the employer. The act, however, does not mandate drug testing.[22] Drug testing and surveillance are guided primarily through state laws.

The ADA and the Civil Rights Act address reference checks and pre-employment physicals. Employee policies should be reviewed by an employment attorney prior to implementation. Employees have certain rights to privacy of their information,[23] so there should be limited access to employee personnel files. In addition, medical files, drug testing (where applicable), and information related to medical conditions and/or bloodborne pathogen exposure should be kept apart and secured away from regular files. Furthermore, any records related to attorney communication about an employee or involving litigation should be retained separately with limited access.[24] Employees should be apprised of the organization policies regarding employee confidentiality at orientation, and these policies should be reinforced regularly with all staff.

Why Have a Security Policy?

To ensure the security of the group practice's property and safety of its employees, employers should develop and maintain a security policy. The best security program cannot function effectively without the support of top management and cooperation of all employees. At the very least, group practices should require employees to wear ID badges to prevent unauthorized entry and possible theft. This allows group practices to identify its employees quickly. The security policy also should note that a member of management is assigned the responsibility of coordinating the group practice's security program.

Issuing keys to employees should be subject to tight security controls. Keys should be issued only with management's approval to employees who need them. Employees should be reminded that keys are medical group property and that they are responsible for safeguarding them. Keys should be returned when an employee is terminated, and before a final paycheck is issued.

When developing policies, the medical practice executive should ensure that security policies are comprehensive. These policies should address violence or potential danger from a variety of sources, including disruptive physicians, visitors, staff, patients, family or friends of staff, and intruders. Systems should be in place to address a variety of situations and, wherever possible, alliances with local law enforcement should be made in advance of an actual emergency. Although it is important for all practices to have a security plan, practices with known risks should regularly perform drills to test proposed policies and procedures. Obvious risk exposures that generate the need for simulation drills include onsite medications, in-office procedures or surgeries, high-risk locations, known substance-abuse or emotionally disturbed patients, and evenings or weekend hours of operation. Clearly, most practices would benefit from a comprehensive security plan and commensurate simulation drills.

It is essential not only to have a plan and policies, but also a staff that is trained, retrained, and continually trained. Emergencies should be rehearsed regularly. Documentation of planning, training, and rehearsal should be maintained.

To be effective, security procedures periodically must be communicated to employees to keep them on security alert.

Emergency/Disaster Guidelines and Drills

It is important to create emergency/disaster plans in order to protect the medical group's employees in time of emergency. Most buildings have fire escape routes posted on the walls, lighted exit signs, and ceiling sprinkler systems; however, these precautions do not protect human life unless specific guidelines and drills are laid out, communicated to all employees, and practiced on a regular basis.

Since September 11, 2001, most employers have seen the need for emergency and disaster plans for both human-made and natural disasters. Policies should be in place directing supervisors and employees on what to do and how to handle emergency situations. Every employee should be notified about all emergency and disaster guidelines during orientation. Drills should be practiced at least once a year, and more frequently if possible. The policies should also direct employees on how to help patients and visitors reach safety.

The practice should have building evacuation plans in case of fire. Whenever an evacuation drill is created, it should include what should happen after the employees get out of the building. Employees should know where to go and to whom to report. Supervisors and managers are appropriate people to put in these types of positions. In an emergency, people generally look to authority figures for direction. Different geographic regions have different threats in terms of natural disasters. In California, for instance, an earthquake emergency plan should be drafted to protect employees. Midwestern states should have a tornado drill. Hurricane-prone areas should have evacuation plans in place for hurricanes and tropical storms.

Every organization should promote "Be Prepared" for disaster programs so employees have emergency provisions and plans for their homes and families.

◢ Federal, State, and Local Laws and Regulations

Not only is it incumbent on employers to be fair and nondiscriminatory in hiring and terminating employees, employers also have a responsibility to provide a safe work environment. A number of laws and regulations apply to protecting personnel. The Fair Labor Standards Act requires employers to pay all nonexempt employees no less than the state minimum wage and requires 1½ times the minimum rate for those who work more than 40 hours a week.[25]

In addition, the Equal Pay Act of 1963 prohibits differences in pay between men and women who perform "substantially equal jobs" unless those differences are due to some factor other than gender, such as merit pay, seniority, or training.[26] These laws refer to the protection of employees from unfair advantage by the employer. Similarly, Title VII of the Civil Rights Act of 1964, which includes actions of sexual harassment, applies not only to the actions of employees and their supervisors, but also to patient interactions with staff, or staff-to-staff interactions. According to the Civil Rights Act, "sexual advances, requests for sexual favors, and other verbal or physical conduct of a sexual nature constitute sexual harassment when this conduct explicitly or implicitly affects an individual's employment, unreasonably interferes with an individual's work performance, or creates an intimidating, hostile, or offensive work environment."[27] This act implies that the employer has a duty to provide protection from psychological harassment or unwanted sexual advances in the workplace.

Through the Americans with Disabilities Act of 1990, the employer is charged with protecting the employee from discrimination because of life impairment that otherwise does not interfere with the ability to perform the job.[28]

◢ Patient Privacy Protection

Policies must include employee responsibility to maintain the confidentiality of patients. Training on the privacy rules of the Health Insurance Portability and Accountability Act of 1996 (HIPAA) should be part of each employee's orientation and repeated regularly. Risk management has revealed that the most frequent violation of patient privacy occurs when the patient is a fellow employee. Because employees have access to medical information through computerized systems, it is tempting for a caring colleague to "check up" on a friend, which violates HIPAA regulations.

Another potential abuse of patient privacy by staff involves the use of computerized information to gather personal information. For example, in one hospital, an employee with an otherwise immaculate record used the computer to locate her estranged husband, who was living with a new partner. In the process, the employee became intrigued with the health status of the husband's new partner, and discovered she was pregnant. The employee lost perspective on the nature of her actions, and when the new partner learned that the employee knew of her condition, she lodged a complaint about breach of privacy. Disciplinary action was taken against the employee, who did not deny the action and was jolted back into recognizing her wrongful activity. Employees must be told and reminded that their right to access information about another person, whether a colleague, family member, or acquaintance, is based on a job-related need to know, and that any other use is a violation of patient privacy.

HIPAA is only one part of patient privacy protection. In many states, the physical presence of a patient on the premises of a health care organization is not, of itself, considered confidential or protected information. This is not true, however, for patients in designated substance abuse treatment programs, who are protected by federal statute,[29] and this is also not true for mental health programs in many states. Regardless of state protection, it is an unwise practice to acknowledge patient presence in the health care office. Unlike an inpatient facility, where the patient has the opportunity to opt out of the patient directory at admission, outpatients are generally not asked their preferences for acknowledgment of their presence. Consequently, it would not be difficult for disgruntled partners, angry acquaintances, estranged spouses, and noncustodial parents to track a potential victim of verbal or physical violence to the physician's office. Staff should be trained to cautiously handle calls from and the physical arrival of such persons. Scripts that do not validate the presence or absence of the patient should be developed and rehearsed. Messages should be taken from the visitor and delivered by staff to the patient, who can then decide whether to allow the person to know of his or her presence in the office. The unanticipated arrival of a spouse or parent bearing a concealed weapon cannot be underestimated. Staff should be trained that patient safety is a priority and that careless management of patient information is grounds for disciplinary action.

Chapter 2 **Managing the Impact of Adverse Legal Events**

THE HEALTH CARE ORGANIZATION is a complex network of exposures. Some exposures can be easily managed and controlled, and some are more insidious. Latent exposures may pass unnoticed until a loss occurs. Furthermore, some exposures are conducive to self-insurance mechanisms, whereas others are better served through commercial insurance. An experienced, qualified insurance broker with expertise in health care is the best counsel to ensure that the organization appropriately addresses financing mechanisms for identified risk exposures.

Insurance Requirements and Products

Each medical practice has its own unique needs. A practice with a great deal of computer equipment might want or need a specific rider to cover that equipment. A practice that has a swimming pool to provide physical therapy may have specific coverage for that. In general, the types of insurance listed below denote the most common types of insurance coverage for a group medical practice:

- Professional liability (medical malpractice);
- General liability;
- Property and casualty;

- Directors and officers liability;

- Workers' compensation (which is not an employee benefit, but a risk control coverage);

- Key person (in small practices);

- Employment liability;

- Environmental;

- Vehicle;

- Helipad (if the organization has one); and

- Business interruption.

The selection of insurance products can be overwhelming. Which product offered by which company will provide the best coverage for the organization's specific needs? Would a self-insured vehicle best meet the organization's financial and exposure needs for all or part of the medical malpractice or workers' compensation coverage? As with any major investment, all parts of the insurance relationship should be evaluated.

Many organizations work with a broker to help procure quotes and make decisions. An insurance broker is different from an agent. An agent represents a single insurance company. Any insurance bought from that individual will be from his or her company. Using an agent may limit the flexibility in coverage that the practice may want. A broker is trained to evaluate the needs of the client and the insurance market. The role of the broker is to find the best coverage for the client's unique needs. Furthermore, the broker has a relationship with the insurers recommended. A broker can negotiate with underwriting to ensure that the client is given the best deal possible for the exposures being insured.

The role of the underwriter is to assess the exposure the health care organization brings to the insurer as the recipient of the risk transfer. The underwriter compares the organization's loss potential with that of similar organizations functioning in similar venues. With that baseline, the underwriter then looks at the specific loss history of the organization to determine the level of risk posed. By using actuarial formulas, the underwriter determines the premium. Other costs are added to the premium based on the insurance company's overhead as well as the services provided by the insurance company.

A skilled broker can also advise the client if self-insurance is in the client's best interest. Working with the broker and an actuary, the organization can conduct a feasibility study. Sometimes the practice will be approaching readiness for self-insurance but is not yet ready to take the leap. A broker can design an interim insurance program that will allow the practice to assume part of the risk before taking the plunge into full self-insurance.

Risk-Benefit Analysis

Even with a skilled broker, the medical practice executive should be prepared to ask questions and to challenge recommendations. To do this, the executive has to have a handle on the risks and benefits of each type of risk-financing vehicle or policy presented. The executive must understand the cost of risk in the organization and have answers to questions about the present coverage such as: What insurance coverage is currently in place? What are the limits of coverage? What are the deductibles, both by claim and aggregate? What are the attachment points for each layer of coverage? What losses have been paid from operations, through loans or through unfunded reserves, during the last five years? Are they losses that should have more formal financing to take advantage of present dollar value?

Once the medical practice executive understands the current cost of coverage, s/he should review the actual practice losses for the last 5 to 10 years. Where did losses occur? Which were the frequent small losses and the less frequent large losses? Were there any unexpected losses? Are there potential losses identified through the risk-assessment process that have not yet occurred but could be devastating to the organization if they should occur? Are there insurance or self-insurance vehicles to prepare for them?

With this information, the executive has a picture of the coverage in place and the exposures that have resulted in losses. The benefits and drawbacks of each type of insurance product must then be weighed. As discussed earlier, the benefit of commercial insurance is that it is known coverage. The limits are defined in the policy, which is a contract of risk transfer between the medical practice and the insurer. The downside of commercial insurance is its overhead and profit loading. The services that are "included" are also included in the premium. Although this might make self-insurance appear to be the only reasonable route, that is not true for every exposure. The cost of some services, such as claims management or risk management, may exceed the rate in the premium. Furthermore, self-insurance requires oversight and administration. The decision to self-insure or to purchase commercial insurance is one of philosophy, convenience, and financial capacity.

▩ Organizational Commitment

Regardless of the type of risk-financing vehicle selected, the organization benefits from tight loss control processes. The temptation to diminish loss control when there is commercial insurance must be avoided. When the insurance market is tight and there is very little competition for customers, those practices with the best loss records and the tightest loss control methods will be the ones with choices regarding an insurer. Those with few processes may find insurance difficult to procure.

Reduction of loss exposure is not just the job of the person with risk management responsibility. It requires commitment on the part of the board and administration to provide the necessary resources for loss control. It further requires that physicians understand the benefit of loss control methods to their practice and that time spent participating in risk management activities may directly relate to less time spent defending their practice in court. Finally, all personnel must realize that risk management is the job of each person in the organization. Although attributed to insurance, true risk management is about people, patients, and staff, as well as maintaining a fiscally viable organization so that the people who work there will continue to have a place to work and to serve others.

◢ Consultative Resources

Every practice has a wealth of internal knowledge and expertise. However, few practices have knowledge and expertise about every business, legal, and financial issue. The business of the medical practice is the delivery of health care. The medical practice executive is charged with having sufficient knowledge to manage the daily operations and with knowing when outside help is required. The use of outside help, however, is costly, but the lack of use of appropriate outside help could be even costlier if an issue is not handled properly.

To develop appropriate professional resources, the medical practice executive must recognize those high-risk areas where outside consultants may be useful. Most often, the areas of business that are complex are fraught with potential for great financial loss, and those that change rapidly and regularly are those for which a resource network is most likely useful. Using that reasoning, such a network would include:

- *Attorneys*. Individual attorneys might be needed for consultation on medical malpractice, employment liability issues, union issues, mergers and acquisitions, tax issues, corporate structure and corporate law, environmental issues, real estate, compliance, workers' compensation, and general corporate concerns.

- *Accountants*. Accountants often specialize in the areas of tax, captive management, foundation management, trusts, Medicare/Medicaid, and other business endeavors.

- *Tax specialists*. Beyond the accountant and attorney are consultants who specialize in tax structures and in maximizing tax advantages. For large organizations or organizations with both nonprofit and for-profit businesses under an umbrella structure, a tax specialist could be a useful consultant.

- *Financial advisors*. Financial advisors assist the organization with making investments that are allowable under Medicare. Medicaid regulations and are in accordance with the practice's corporate and tax structure.

■ *Insurance brokers.* An experienced insurance broker is essential for ensuring that the organization develops a comprehensive risk-financing program that addresses the known exposures. The organization may choose to use the services of one broker, or it may have multiple brokers for different lines of coverage expertise.

■ *Environmental consultants.* Although the practice may have appropriate mechanisms for disposal of hazardous waste and may not incinerate or generate gases, there may still be environmental concerns related to assumption of responsibility for previous owners of the property or for the environmental impact of new construction. An environmental consultation is sometimes recommended when participating in a merger or acquisition or in a divestment of property.

The need for consultants changes with the needs of the organization. Because this is a fluid area, it is important that the medical practice executive be clear about recruiting, working with, and retaining experts. Due diligence on the credentials and credibility of consultants is highly recommended.

■ Contract Negotiations with Consultants

The medical practice executive must be clear about the level of expertise it expects and requires for the job to be done. The contract should clearly state the medical practice's expectations about the nature and level of expertise to be provided. In addition, contracts should clearly state the amount and type of service to be delivered and the expected time frame for deliverables. Consultants will generally attempt to shift all liability for outcome to the medical practice under the rationale that it ultimately decides how much of the consultant's advice to implement. It is important that the contract be reviewed carefully to ensure that there is not an undue burden being placed on the practice to accept liability for acts of the consultant over which it has no control. In the end, the medical practice executive must weigh the risks of consultant use against the benefits. Although costly to use, the time, energy, and expertise gained through outsourcing complex high-risk activities may outweigh the cost and the headache.[30]

Current and Future Risk-Related Issues

Often the resource network consists of relationships that are activated on an as-needed basis. Rather than entering into single contract projects, the practice may choose to have certain consultants on retainer, or may choose to have periodic interactions between contractual projects. These types of relationships frequently emerge naturally with time and positive working encounters. Nevertheless, the practice may desire to cultivate certain relationships based on its specific needs. Recognition of past needs for specialists in communication, medical records, or information systems may generate a need to maintain ongoing relationships with consultants in any given area. For example, a current litigation may awaken the practice to realize that the high-risk birth program has some unaddressed exposures. Perhaps the risk assessment of the patient flow process demonstrates areas of latent exposure to communication breakdown that could lead to a system failure, medical error, and patient injury. Consultant relationships can improve the practice's operation when the consultant fits the organization's culture and philosophical approach to health care.

Contract Negotiation

Contract negotiation is a complex activity. Contracts create legally binding obligations between two parties. Every contract is unique and requires careful consideration. The nature of the contract dictates the components that are most critical. Contracts with payers will focus on protection of public health information, agreed amount of payment, time frame for payment, billing procedures, accessibility to other records, risk transfer, and more. Contracts with physicians, however, will be significantly different. With a physician the practice is concerned about level of expertise and the maintenance of that expertise, the amount of work, and the nature of the work, as well as agreed-upon compensation.

Issues such as benefits and compensation plan contingencies will be a large component of the contract, as may noncompete clauses or other business agreements. Transfer of risk may not be an issue if the practice is going to provide professional liability insurance. If such insurance is not provided by the practice, the contract should specify the amount of expected coverage and the frequency for providing proof of insurance. With contractors and vendors, the terms are often more concrete. The deliverables are usually goods or specific services and the issues of transfer of risk are even greater. Some specific components are critical to all contracts:

- Parties are named;

- Expectations for performance are delineated;

- The length of the contract and the date of its termination are stipulated;

- The insurance requirements and indemnification requirements are delineated;

- How the contract gets amended is specified;

- The choice of law governing the contract is defined; and

- Whether the contract can be assigned is addressed.

Other provisions might include review of records, any exhibits or appendices, and conditions for alternative dispute resolution.[31]

◢ Health Care Law

All contracts entered into by the practice should be reviewed to ensure they comply with applicable health care laws. Practices that accept federal funds need to be particularly careful that no conditions of participation or regulations applicable to recipients of federal monies are violated. Physicians must be educated about the implications of Stark I and II and the antikickback laws. In addition, legal counsel should be queried not only about the contract conditions themselves, but also whether the contract sets up any potential conflicts that could be seen as antitrust, Stark, or antikick-back violations.

The medical practice as an entity is not the only party at risk. Through peer discussion and education by legal counsel, physician members of the practice group need to understand the implications of their personal investment in companies that might be perceived as creating a Stark or other legal conflict with their role in the practice. No business contract related to health care services should be entered by either the organization or its member physicians without a careful review by legal counsel to avoid complicated allegations of improper acts.

■ Needs Assessment

Contracts are binding legal documents, and as such they should not be considered lightly. If a contract is not necessary, perhaps there are situations in which it should be avoided. Contract negotiation is a skill. The more experience the medical practice executive accumulates, the more astute s/he will become at identifying potential exposures created through contractual language. The medical practice executive bearing the risk management responsibility should consider:

- The organization's past contractual experience – whether with a potential contractor or with others;

- The present situation – whether it warrants a contractual agreement or if it could be best served in another way;

- The future needs of the organization – whether this is a long-term relationship that might be better served as an employment relationship or if this need is a short-term one that warrants a limited relationship;

- The competitive advantages to having this relationship – whether the practice gains knowledge, expertise, or a unique approach; and

- The trends in the field – whether using this service is going to move the organization toward its long-term competitive goals.

■ Risk Management Strategy

Risk management is a process, not a function. As such, the medical practice executive's perspective and focus on risk management depends on his or her belief system, values, and perceived organizational relative exposure. Nevertheless, for risk management to be effective, there should be a plan and a strategy to ensure that exposures are adequately identified and addressed.

There are many approaches to a risk management plan; however, certain elements are universal to all plans:

- Exposures should be addressed in the key areas of patient care, medical staff, employee relations, financial risks, property risks, and technological risks. Other types of risks the organization may have are technical, vehicular, and environmental. Any key area of the organization's operation should be addressed.[32]

- A system should be in place for financing potential losses.

- The board and leadership should be knowledgeable about exposures and losses and should be engaged in prevention.[33]

Although this volume has reinforced the notion that risk management is a comprehensive activity that includes all elements of the organization's function and processes, it remains true that the greatest exposure for significant ongoing financial loss for a health care organization is in the area of medical malpractice.

Given that, the strategy to address injury to patients is key to a successful risk management program. In patient care, as in every other aspect of the organization, the most effective way to control loss is to prevent it. That is the goal. Because of human variability and the vast number of services and procedures provided by medical organizations, however, it will be many years before all the latent errors currently in existence can be adequately addressed. By then, more errors will have emerged with the proliferation of new technologies, medications, and procedures.

A successful risk management plan must include a method to constantly monitor new exposures and address existing exposures in patient care. Staff should be included in the process in whatever ways are reasonable. The most basic level is reporting actual and potential errors. Every potential error is an opportunity to prevent a loss in the future because it exposes a latent failure in the system. Reporting systems that include near misses or potential loss events are key to an effective risk management plan. Other tools for assessment include loss runs from previous claims, surveys and assessment tools, and reports from outside consultants.

Reporting is not limited to situations of human error or process, however. It includes malfunction of medical devices, which include any device that is not a medication used in the process of treatment – from simple tongue depressors up through the most complex equipment. The Safe Medical Devices Act of 1990 (SMDA) requires that device users notify the manufacturer, or the Food and Drug Administration if the manufacturer is not known, about any malfunction that involves serious injury or death of a patient.[34] Often the malfunction of medical devices is attributed by health care workers to "user error," or a work-around provides temporary remediation of the problem. In an effective risk management program, users are encouraged to report all events, including the duct taping of hoses or alarms that do not trigger, in an effort to forestall medical events that may be device related. If equipment is involved in a claim, it should be impounded. Under no circumstances should it be repaired or returned to the manufacturer. It is key evidence should the claim proceed to litigation.

Peer review activity as a process for improving care is essential. Peer review activities, appropriately carried out, identify variability in the practice, which leads to less reliability in the system. It can also point out those providers who consistently achieve better than average results as well as those outliers who may require assistance. Peer review should not be used as a cloak to avoid transparency and truthfulness with patients. It should be used as intended – for physicians to monitor their peers to ensure and achieve a higher level of medical practice and care for patients.

Finally, the risk management strategy should include the organization's philosophy about claims management and investigation. Immediate investigation of a claim provides the best defense against fading memory and alteration or disappearance of evidence. In addition, early investigation provides the opportunity to identify the latent failures in the system that led to at least one patient injury, and could, if unaddressed, soon lead to another. Care should be taken to ensure that all discussions about the claim are protected under attorney direction as part of the claims investigation process. All original medical records should be locked so that no changes can be made to them. A copy of the record should be made and put into circulation for the continuing care of the patient.

The SMDA has limited application in the office practice setting. For example, physician practices are exempt from the law, whereas ambulatory surgery centers and outpatient diagnostic and treatment facilities (e.g., chemotherapy and dialysis) must comply with it.[35] The professional in charge of risk management should be aware of the appropriate application for the setting in which care is being provided.

Chapter 3 **Establishing a Plan for Disaster Response and Recovery**[36]

DISASTER RECOVERY PLANNING has been a required function for corporate America since the early 1990s. This planning encompasses all functions within an organization and is designed to deal with a wide range of problems from a minor disruption in service delivery such as a short-term loss of electricity to major disasters like Hurricane Katrina.

Although medical practice administrators have taken care to back up computer systems, they have little or no training in disaster recovery or business continuity planning. In the past few years, these professionals have been faced with the challenge of recovering from tumultuous events, both natural and human-made, which have resulted in serious business interruptions. In some cases these disasters have threatened the very survival of the practice.

The medical practice administrator is the individual who will be expected to carry out the process of putting the organization back on its feet, both during and after a disaster hits. However, disaster recovery planning training has not been included on most curricula offered to practice administrators. Nor do these busy individuals have the time to review the extensive literature available to help devise a workable solution for their individual organizations.

This chapter presents a synopsis of disaster recovery and business continuity planning guidelines. In addition, it identifies some critical processes that should be included in a disaster recovery plan prepared for a physician office practice.

Using a combination of personal experience and extensive literature review, this author will present information that will validate the need for a comprehensive disaster recovery/business continuity plan in the physician office practice. This is the first step in alerting the practice stakeholders that time and resources should be allotted to this valuable tool.

Additionally, this chapter provides a framework to help practice managers identify mission-critical processes and present suggested time frames to get these processes back on line, ensuring the economic survival of the organization. This will be accomplished by reviewing the procedures used in the business community and modifying them to work within a physician practice.

Included in this discussion will be a review of both liability issues as well as insurance needs resulting from a business interruption caused by an untoward event.

Although plans will differ among practices, a road map will assist the medical practice executive to identify many of their mission-critical processes and help determine the appropriate action to be taken in the event of a disaster.

▚ What Is a Disaster?

There are a number of definitions for a disaster. It can be "an event which causes loss of an essential service or part of it for a length of time which imperils business,"[37] or "a calamitous event, especially one occurring suddenly and causing great loss of life, damage or hardship as a flood, airplane crash or business failure."[38] In other words a disaster is an event that makes normal functions impossible.

Disasters can be natural or human-made. Witness the destruction caused by Hurricane Katrina and the subsequent flooding of

New Orleans in 2005, or the Arizona wildfires in the spring of 2006. Human-made disasters can be work stoppages such as the recent transit strikes in Philadelphia and New York or the destruction caused by terrorist attacks on the World Trade Center in 2001.

Tornadoes, fires, electrical storms, and chemical spills all have the power to damage critical supply lines and make it impossible for a medical practice to function on a normal level. What would happen to a practice if a pipe in an office above were to rupture, pouring water onto the server or file room?

When does an operational incident escalate to a disaster? In the summer of 2004, what initially looked like a tripped circuit breaker in one medical practice office was recognized to be a blackout that affected the entire city of New York. In 2006 the electric company prevented a recurrence by advising customers to go to generator power or risk another area-wide loss of electricity. While both incidents required that critical systems such as servers be powered off, the former mandated putting a disaster plan into force to assist with the safe evacuation of personnel, either getting them home or to a local area shelter for the evening.

New Orleans thought it had weathered the worst of Hurricane Katrina until the reality of the broken levees devastated the city. Plans put in place for a one- to three-day incident escalated overnight into a true full-blown disaster that was still evolving a year later.[39]

How does a medical practice plan for this type of calamity? These incidents are rare, but the economic impact on the practices affected can be staggering. It is estimated that "30 percent of companies that suffer a catastrophic disaster never get back to business and another 29 percent close within two years of the disaster."[40] Employers look to their medical practice executives and expect they will provide leadership in this vital area of medical practice administration and oversight.

There are numerous Websites, articles, and textbooks written in the past few years that will document how to prepare a disaster recovery/business continuity plan. The best practices from this literature search have been pulled together in this chapter and the plans have been refined to make them workable in a medical practice environment.

◢ What Is a Disaster Recovery Plan?

Disaster recovery planning has often been associated with information technology functions. If a network, server, or personal computer goes down, how does one ensure that the data is recoverable and how quickly can the system get back on line? Because a vast majority of practices today rely on practice management software for appointments and billing functions, medical practice administrators have a working knowledge of the steps needed to repair systems and recover data.

However, the medical practice executive needs to review the entire business in light of this type of planning. If there is no access to the facility and the doctors cannot treat patients, there is no revenue. If there is no access to the bank, the practice is unable to process payroll or pay bills – or deposit additional funds. If there is no telephone service, how do patients get in touch with the practice for emergencies, appointments, or questions about follow up?

A disaster plan consists of precautions to be taken so that effects of a disaster will be minimized and the organization can resume mission-critical functions. This planning can be divided into a six-stage cycle. The stages are risk assessment, business impact analysis, business continuity strategy development, business continuity plan development, testing, and maintenance.[41]

◢ Risk Assessment

When performing a risk assessment, it is important not only to look at how the risk might affect the practice but also to look at the likelihood of the threat. Although there is a geologic fault running along 14th Street in New York City, it is not the San Andreas Fault. Disaster planning for earthquakes in New York would rank very low on the likelihood scale compared to areas in California and the West Coast. Depending on the area of the country, an office practice can be affected by hurricanes, tornadoes, blizzards, floods, and electrical storms, to name a few natural disasters. Even extremes of temperature might have an adverse effect on business, not to mention the threat of a flu pandemic.

Internal Control: Guidance for Directors on the Combined Code (also known as the Turnbull Report), published by the Internal Central Working Party of the Institute of Chartered Accountants in England and Wales, provides guidance on the implementation of internal controls enabling companies to identify and respond to changing risks, both internal and external. The corporate governance codes recommended in this report published in 1999 are now being established worldwide.[42]

These codes help examine the financial, business, compliance, and operational areas of the business and rank the potential risks as high impact/high likelihood, high impact/low likelihood, low impact/high likelihood, and low impact/low likelihood.[43] Ranking the perceived risks using this methodology, one would be able to put time and effort into projects that could potentially have a significant impact on a medical practice. It is also possible that the final plan may consist of a number of smaller plans allowing several issues to be addressed once and inserted into various disaster recovery plan scenarios. For example, a practice could set up miniature disaster recovery plans to cope with problems such as loss of electricity (local and systemwide), loss of computers (systemwide), loss of phones/T1/DSL lines (local and systemwide), and loss of a transportation network and in doing so would have identified many issues required in most disaster recovery plans.

▰ Business Impact Analysis

In addition to reviewing potential risks, it is also imperative to take a look at key performance indicators: the people, the knowledge, and the equipment that allow a practice to function on a day-to-day basis. If any of these three elements are missing, the practice cannot function at its optimum level. There are a number of ways to gather this information. One can send out a survey to various departments or to the individuals responsible for that office function. One can also meet with and interview these individuals one on one. Both of these methods have been found lacking in gathering accurate and reliable data.

The most effective method of gathering this critical information is usually a combination of a survey followed by a group meeting across all functions. This allows personnel to agree to own a process, recognize the impact of a disaster on the individual department or function, and agree to the steps that need to be taken to get the functions back on line. For example, coding books might be used by the physicians, the checkout personnel, as well as billing personnel. However, billing personnel would probably consider this a critical need while the physicians and other personnel might be focused on ways to contact patients regarding appointments, and so on.

During the discussions of impact analysis, the question of moving to an alternate site may arise. Disaster recovery plans refer to sites as hot, warm, and cold. A hot site is one that is a total standby environment. Unless the practice has an office in another location, on a different power grid and serviced by a different telephone provider, the expense of maintaining this type of site would be prohibitive. A warm site is a standby environment lacking only those requirements that can be provided quickly. For example, if there is a loss of power to one area of the building and a conference room is set up with additional phone and computer cabling powered by generator, it could be utilized in this emergency situation. A cold site is a standby location without any hardware available.[44] Without the luxury of having a second office as a backup, smaller practices would be forced to a cold site if access to the office is prohibited for any period of time.

◢ Strategy and Plan Development

Once the impact analysis is completed and there is a clearer understanding of the practice's critical processes, it is time to develop the strategy and plan for getting these functions back on line. The plan must clearly identify the tasks that need to be accomplished along with the timeline for progress. It is also imperative that the personnel responsible for these tasks be identified as well as the location(s) used; that is, alternate office, home, cold site, and so forth.

These plans must be as detailed as possible if they are to be effective. Sit at a desk with only a computer and a phone and attempt to do a day's work. Within a very short time, one would recognize the little things that are used every day and taken for granted; that is, stapler, pen, pencil, sticky notes, and so on.

It is also important that the methods and procedures for bringing back these critical processes be documented in the event the persons responsible have been adversely affected by the disaster and are unable to complete their task. Plans should cover the possibility that personnel may have other commitments if the disaster is wide ranging. They may have friends and family affected by the disaster. They may be responsible for the care of young children or elderly, sick relatives. If staff members have no access to money or transportation, they may be unable to get to work to assist with disaster recovery efforts.

◢ Plan Testing and Maintenance

After the plan has been developed, it is critical that it be tested. Again, the literature demonstrates that only about 40 percent of disaster plans are actually tested. Of the plans that are tested, 80 percent fail in one or more areas. However, that failure is perceived as a positive number, because the corrections are made during the testing stage and not discovered in the middle of an actual disaster.

The testing is often the most difficult part of the planning process. Most experts in the field recommend testing part of the plan, in short intervals in case of plan failure. The only time a full-scale disaster drill should be called is when one is assured that all elements will function perfectly.[45]

◢ Critical Processes

After reviewing the outline for developing a disaster recovery plan, it is time to look at some critical processes that would be similar in almost all medical office practices, no matter the size or the specialty. These processes include evacuation, communication, finances, insurance claims, human resources, clinical concerns, servers and information systems, telecommunications, and the physical plant.

Evacuation

To ensure against liability, it is important to remember that employers owe statutory and common-law duties of care to employees: "…officers of the company may be personally held liable to pay compensation for incidents relating to the safety of the company's product and environmental damage."[46] Common sense also warns that if the building is unsafe due to fire, loss of electrical power, or any other reason, there should be a plan to safely evacuate staff, patients, and visitors.

If an evacuation needs to be implemented and there are patients and friends in the office, have the clinical staff assume the responsibility to escort them to the emergency exits and assist them to take the stairs. In an emergency, particularly a fire, do not use the elevators. Assign one member of the reception/front desk staff to check all exam rooms to ensure all patients have been evacuated.

When a room has been evacuated, the door should be closed as a visual cue that the room check has been completed. However if, as in many practices, a closed door means the room is occupied, a different visual cue needs to be used. One suggestion is to take the pillow from the exam table and place it outside the closed door.

Additionally, in the event that the practice will not be able to gain access to the premises for a period of time, it will be prudent to ensure that all deposits and mail containing checks be removed at the time of the evacuation along with current encounters and chart notes.

If time allows, the servers should be powered down, the previous days' backup tapes taken, and phones forwarded to the answering service.

The person designated as the team leader for an evacuation should check the premises to ensure that all patients, friends, and staff have departed. Additionally, as part of the disaster recovery plan, the staff should meet at a preordained area to ensure that all staff have evacuated and can be accounted for. At this time, further instructions can be delivered to the staff.

The plan should include the possibility that the staff was evacuated without checkbooks, credit cards, cell phones, wallets, or keys. Are there working flashlights available in case there is a loss of electricity and there are no lights in the hallways and stairwells? Since 9/11, some New Yorkers have kept small personal-sized flashlights attached to the lanyards holding their identification (ID) tags.

Communication

It is imperative that lines of communication be set up with staff, patients, and vendors as soon as possible after a disaster. The practice administrator or designee should have an employee contact list with home and cellular telephone numbers as well as e-mail addresses. If an employee is hurt during an evacuation, the practice will need emergency contact information. Is that readily available? Where is this information stored – on a computer in the office that is now unavailable?

How will the practice contact patients? Does off-site backup data contain patient names and phone numbers and how can this data be accessed if servers are not available? Can the answering service act as a backup call center to make necessary phone calls while the office is inaccessible?

How can the practice contact vendors to let them know of the emergency and perhaps place orders for replacement equipment. Where are contact numbers stored? What about account numbers, passwords, and other essential information that a medical practice executive always has available "at their fingertips" when in the office?

More importantly, how can physicians, staff, and vendors get in touch with the practice administrator? Again, look to the answering service to see if they are able to set up a call center to forward messages to a cell phone, an e-mail address, and so forth.

In the event of an impending disaster such as a hurricane and if an evacuation occurs in a widespread area over a number of days, it is critical to have updated employee contact information. If the area is evacuating, having an employee's home number will not be sufficient and cell phones may be off line for a period of time.

Finances

One of the most critical areas to plan for in a disaster is finances. If the office is closed and there are no patient appointments booked, there is an immediate affect on cash flow. If the practice does not participate in electronic funds transfer from all payers and the mail cannot be delivered, cash flow is affected.

If there has been an area-wide evacuation and the bank is now unavailable, how does the practice access its accounts? If the evacuation only affected the main office, do any of the satellite offices have access to all the contact information, checkbooks, and deposit slips needed to access the account for deposits and withdrawals?

How will payroll be processed? Are there sufficient funds to cover? Does the practice have business interruption insurance? What does it cover, for how long, and what are the limitations? If the practice is shut down for a period of time, which employees will be paid? Does a decision to not pay employees affect their health insurance coverage?

Are copies of managed care contracts, particularly those with carve-out reimbursements, stored in an off-site facility? Is insurance contact information available so payers can be alerted and possibly avoid denials due to untimely filing during this emergency period?

Insurance Claims

Is the information regarding the practice insurance carriers available off site?

Commercial insurance covers buildings and contents, whereas business interruption insurance is meant to cover the incremental costs incurred through dislocation. Business interruption insurance does not cover the full cost of getting the practice back to normal working conditions. When formulating a disaster recovery plan, the practice administrator should meet with the insurance carriers and discuss their requirements for damage documentation, their response times, and any limitations on policies. Other questions that should be asked of the carrier include whether salvage can begin before an adjuster arrives. Will they believe a molten lump of metal was an expensive server destroyed by fire?[47]

Video and still cameras can be used to document damage. All damaged materials should be kept on site until an adjustor releases. The insurance carrier should be asked how the replacement value of an item is determined. Because the practice will need cash to get back on its feet, it is important to know how quickly claims will be paid.

If the untoward event was caused by a terrorist attack, is there coverage under the current policy or is it excluded under the "act of war" clause? It is also important to be aware that property/casualty companies are increasingly reluctant to write policies covering disaster recovery in certain areas of the country.

Human Resources

The most valued resource for a practice is the staff. It is critical that their needs be reviewed and addressed as part of any successful disaster recovery plan. If the disaster has affected a wide area, such as New York City's transit strike in December 2005, there are employee issues that need to be resolved. Employees who lived in New Jersey and Long Island could get to Manhattan and walk to work. Those who lived in the outer boroughs like Brooklyn, Queens, and the Bronx could only get to work by car. However, parking was limited and the city mandated multiple riders in autos coming into Manhattan.

In order to staff the office, carpools were set up, schedules were flexed, and the work day was shortened. This permitted the office to remain open assisting the patient population while addressing the needs of the staff during a time of crisis.

In situations like this, the practice administrator should consider rewarding those employees who can work longer hours rather than punish those who, because of family commitments, cannot come in earlier or stay later to work through an emergency.

Consider having photo IDs for employees. If there is an untoward event in the building or area, law enforcement may refuse entrance to those without the proper credentials.

If the untoward event will deny access to the facility for a period of time, it is important to have license and credentialing information available for the clinical staff.

The most important element for handling human resource issues during a time of disaster is to communicate, plan, and involve.

Clinical Concerns

How can the practice communicate with patients if there is no access to the office? Is there capability to remotely forward the practice phone lines? If yes, who knows the passwords and number required to do so? Where is this information kept?

How will the practice handle ongoing patient care? Is there a physician office or hospital area where patients can be seen for a few hours a day? Do the physicians require any special equipment? If yes, this equipment will need to be stocked in the standby facility.

How will physicians access patient records? If the practice uses an electronic medical record and has an off-site backup, how quickly can access be restored?

For those practices with paper records, not only is access delayed, but many disasters such as hurricanes and flooding can destroy paper records. Wet paper begins to deteriorate in three hours. However, it is important to note that paper documents, unless water soluble inks were used, can be recovered from water damage. If the documents cannot be immediately recovered, they should be frozen with dry ice. The atmosphere in the room should be stabilized to 50 to 60 degrees with the humidity at 25 to 35 percent. Metal fasteners should be removed to prevent rust from running onto the paper; no attempts should be made to separate papers when they are wet.[48] There are a number of vendors that specialize in recovery of water-damaged documents and books. Consider contacting them to see what their response time would be when establishing a disaster recovery plan.

It is also important to remember that during disasters, the practice is still required to maintain the privacy and security of both medical and financial records under the Health Insurance Portability and Accountability Act guidelines. One should not be tempted to indiscriminately toss out those wet, moldy paper files.

Servers and Information Systems

This is probably the one area of disaster recovery that most practices have already addressed. Daily backups and redundant systems are the norm in today's practices. Can employees working in remote locations have the ability to access the practice network? That would allow certain employees like billers to work from home for a period of time while the facility was not available.

Practices that utilize an application service provider (ASP) may have access to their data more quickly because the data and servers are off site and possibly outside of the affected disaster area. However, it is important to investigate the ASP's disaster plans and ensure access to the practice data if they have a disruptive event on their site.

Telecommunications

Telephones are a practice's lifeline to the outside world. However, today's phones are usually attached to computer systems, which means that a loss of power means phones are not available. This became very apparent when New York was hit with a power blackout in 2004. The practice should have one single-user corded phone for just such an emergency. Most offices have at least one line that does not go through their private branch exchange. It could be the fax line, a modem, or the line used for credit card transactions. Plugging a corded phone into that line will at least allow the practice to make outgoing calls to the answering service and to remotely transfer calls to a working number.

Consider how important it might be to have the practice's answering service/call center located in a different power grid and telephone service area. This way, the call center might still be up and running and able to handle the practice's additional call volume. The call center must also have its own disaster recovery plan in place, which should be reviewed by the practice.

If systems are up and running but access to the site is being denied, program the message reminder system remotely and change the outgoing messages to alert patients of the problem.

Physical Plant

When the practice can again gain access to the physical plant, the first priority is to contain the damage. Save everything that can be salvaged and restored and keep the damaged equipment for the adjustor to review. Be sure to have an up-to-date fixed inventory list accessible. The age and purchase price of the destroyed equipment will need to be documented. Copies of receipts will speed the turn-around time on claims.

Research the vendors who can respond quickly to assess and contain fire and water damage. Keep those names with the contact information for insurance claims. Items may look unrecoverable, but salvage must be started immediately to prevent rust, corrosion, and mold.

Keep a contact list of all vendors and make video or photo records of the damage incurred. It may be quicker to replace equipment instead of restoring, but it's usually more expensive. Restoring avoids capital expenditure and improves cash flow. This might be critical because the insured value may be less than the cost of replacement and it may take months to process claims.

If there is no access to the plant for a period of time and the doctors and staff will be practicing at a remote location, be sure it is equipped with all the necessary equipment. Think about copier, fax, stamps, desk supplies, stationery, and prescription pads in addition to fax and phones.

■ Critical Process Time Frames

After the critical processes for the practice have been established, the next step is to determine how quickly these need to be up and running. First, determine the:

- Maximum tolerable downtime – the maximum time an organization can tolerate being down;

- Recovery time objective – the time available to recover;

- Recovery point objective (RPO) – the extent of data lost; and

- Work recovery time (WRT) – the time available to recover data.

Critical process time frames are usually set at (1) 24 hours, (2) three to five days, (3) one to two weeks, and (4) one to two months. Prior to Hurricane Katrina, these time frames worked for most disasters. For example, a practice would want to set the critical process time frame for getting telephones back on line at 24 hours.

Although the practice may also want access to servers and computers within 24 hours, the RPO and WRT may be two or three days. These time frames should be reviewed carefully and should be realistic. Think of alternative ways to solve the problem. Set up workaround solutions (i.e., use paper until the systems are back on line).

Be aware that staff may need to function in different capacities during this time period. Some of the staff may be focused on damage control and recovery. Other staff members may be required to take all the information that had been worked on paper and enter this backlog into the computers when they are back on line. Additionally, other staff may be handling the day-to-day functions of the office.

Put together a matrix list of employees and their various skills in order to ensure that the right people with the right skills are assigned to these critical functions.

Along with detailing the time frames to get processes up and running, it is critical that the practice administrator reviews when staff should return to work. Time frames should be set for when the practice's billing, administrative, clinical, and ancillary staff should return. For example, if the physical therapy unit will not be ready to see patients for 30 days, then there is no reason for the physical therapy staff to be standing around the office with nothing to do. Can they fill in with other duties?

Completed Plan

Once the disaster plan is completed, it will be necessary to test it. As stated previously, it is better to run smaller tests of specific areas of the plan rather than a complete disaster drill.

The plan should be reviewed annually and updated as needed. When staff are hired (or terminated), the plan need to be updated to reflect those changes. Employee contact information should be updated every six months, as individuals frequently change cell phones and acquire new numbers. The plan and all changes should be communicated to all employees of the practice. In New York, plans are reviewed with staff whenever the terror alert changes, a frequent occurrence in 2004 and 2005.

Summary

Disaster recovery/business continuity planning is a critical function overlooked by many medical practice executives. Although it is time-consuming to review the risks and critical processes within a practice, it is also an excellent time to review how procedures actually work. It also presents an opportunity to get feedback from the staff that actually performs the jobs.

Although no one expects to use a disaster recovery plan, having one in place will help in the first minutes and hours when the disaster plan is invoked. Personnel will know their jobs, which helps to keep the staff calm and focused on the problem at hand.

This chapter highlights the critical areas to consider when developing a disaster recovery plan. However, because each practice differs in its mission and philosophy, only a practice manager with a working knowledge of how the practice functions can create a complete and effective disaster recovery plan.

Chapter 4 **Developing and Implementing a Compliance Program for Federal and State Laws and Regulations**

◼ Contract Law

Recipients of federal monies must comply with specific laws related to the reporting of activity, the nature of contractual relationships, and the regulations pertaining to employees and employment. A prudent risk management strategy involves working with an attorney familiar with federal contracting requirements. In addition, the medical practice executive should strive to keep abreast of the most current information provided through the Centers for Medicare and Medicaid Services (CMS) and other information sources. CMS provides regular updates for physicians and health care organizations. In addition, Web subscriptions, such as Government Policy Newslinks,[49] scan all federal publications daily searching for changes and significant postings. These scanning services send out a daily link to all important information. Although there is a significant amount of information not directly related to government contracting, other types of pertinent health care information, including the *Federal Register*, provide the medical practice executive with up-to-date information on trends.

Federal, State, and Local Laws and Regulations

In addition to law specific to contracts, other state, federal, and local laws influence compliance. The purpose of compliance programs is to ensure adherence to federal regulation. Although they apply to the organization's relationship with employees, Occupational Safety and Health Administration regulations, the Family Medical Leave Act, and the Americans with Disabilities Act are all part of the corporate compliance program. Consequently, compliance with these regulations is implied in the acceptance of federal funds.

Safe and Secure: How to Create an Effective OSHA Compliance Program in Your Practice[50]

Medical group practice administrators have a responsibility to provide a safe working environment for their employees and patients. The federal Occupational Safety and Health Administration (OSHA), either directly or through designated state agencies, develops safety standards and ensures compliance with those standards for virtually all employers in the health care industry. Every practice needs to create, implement, and document an OSHA compliance plan that encompasses:

- Exit routes, emergency action plans, and fire prevention plans;
- Hazardous materials;
- Personal protective equipment;
- Medical and first aid;
- Fire protection;
- Compressed gases;
- Electrical;

- Toxic and hazardous substances; and
- Needlestick safety.

The practice administrator must recognize that OSHA can levy citations and fines for noncompliance with its standards.

Designate an OSHA Safety Officer

The administrator will need to designate an employee as the OSHA safety officer. In smaller groups, the administrator may need to assume this role. An employee with a clinical background can also be appropriate. The safety officer is responsible for:

- Developing and maintaining the OSHA safety program and procedure manual for the facility;
- Training all new employees in the safety standards;
- Reviewing the OSHA safety program annually for all employees;
- Meeting record-keeping requirements;
- Conducting annual reviews of the safety standards adopted by the facility; and
- Representing the facility in the event of an inspection by an OSHA compliance safety and health officer.

The safety officer will evaluate and recommend the adoption of standards and procedures for the medical group. It is imperative that the organization provides strong support to the safety officer and that group leaders recognize the importance of the OSHA safety program. The program should be adopted as a component of the group's compliance efforts.

Consider the Physical Environment

Medical practice administrators should consider the overall physical environment when evaluating compliance issues under OSHA's general duty clause. Obvious elements of a compliance program that address this clause include:

- Review of the facility's physical space, including air quality, floor and wall openings, exiting or egress (including evacuation), exit doors and signs, adequate lighting, storage areas, stairs and stairways, and elevated surfaces;

- Evaluation of fire safety, including sprinkler systems, fire alarms, fire and evacuation procedures, fire drills, and the availability and use of fire extinguishers;

- Review of electrical safety procedures, including annual inspection of electrical devices, cords, grounding of electrical circuits and lockout/tagout of machinery, equipment, and circuits as appropriate; and

- Determination of proper installation, training, and use of automated external defibrillators as appropriate.

In addition, a medical practice must comply with OSHA standards for emergency action, personal protective equipment, fire protection, bloodborne pathogens, hazard communications, and tuberculosis control.

Commitment Is Staffwide

The commitment to creating standards for workplace safety should begin with physicians but requires buy-in from all levels of staff to create a meaningful compliance program. To demonstrate management's commitment and to achieve facilitywide involvement, OSHA recommends:[51]

- Posting a statement of policy on worker safety and health next to the OSHA workplace poster;

- Holding meetings to communicate the group's commitment to safety and to discuss objectives for safety and health;

- Involving the administrator in facility assessments and reviews of incident reports to ensure that appropriate follow-up occurs;

- Following facility policy at all times;

- Involving employees in setting safety procedures, conducting training, and investigating accidents to make use of their specialized knowledge and increasing their buy-in;

- Including assignments of safety responsibility as part of the employees' job descriptions;

- Including compliance with safety policies and procedures in employee evaluations; and
- Annually reviewing safety objectives and reevaluating the need for compliance program revisions or new objectives.

Service Available for Assessment

The medical practice administrator is responsible for knowing what is needed to meet employee and patient safety in the facility. OSHA maintains a consultation service that will provide information about potential hazards and methods to improve workplace safety. The program is targeted to smaller businesses and is separate from the OSHA inspection program. In evaluating potential deficiencies in meeting OSHA standards, the consultation does not issue citations or penalties, and the confidential findings are not routinely reported to OSHA inspection staff. Every state and U.S. territory has an OSHA consultation office.

Mitigate Workplace Hazards

To mitigate hazards in the workplace, OSHA suggests that medical practices:

- Establish safe work procedures and ensure that employees follow them;
- Be prepared to enforce rules with an appropriate disciplinary system;
- Provide personal protective equipment, where appropriate, and train employees in its use and proper maintenance;
- Plan for emergencies, including regular drills; and
- Make appropriate arrangements for employees to have access to medical personnel for advice and response to illness or injuries.

Employee Training Imperative

Employee training should create knowledge of materials and equipment, the known and potential hazards that may exist in the workplace, and how to control or minimize those hazards. No employee should undertake a job until he or she has been properly trained to perform it, nor undertake a job that appears unsafe or in which potential hazards have not been minimized. Training should include both instruction and demonstration by qualified personnel, such as laboratory or phlebotomy supervisors on the use of sharps, fire department personnel on the use of fire extinguishing equipment, and radiation safety officers on the use of dosimetry badges and lead gowns. Practices can also use Web-based broadcasts on safety-related topics.

All new employees need to receive training on the general standards of the facility (e.g., fire and evacuation procedures) and job-specific hazards. Staff should have additional training when changes in the work environment alter potential or actual safety hazards. A medical practice should provide annual training on all aspects of the safety compliance program. Documentation of this training should include a listing and signatures of the employees present, the date, the type of training, the subjects covered in the training, the person performing the training and his or her credentials.

These points are the basis for the creation and implementation of the OSHA compliance plan for a medical group practice. The OSHA *Small Business Handbook* provides a thorough primer (see "OSHA Website Resources").

State and Local Compliance Is Required

The Occupational Safety and Health Act encourages states and territorial jurisdictions to develop and operate their own safety enforcement programs. These programs are approved and monitored by OSHA, which provides up to 50 percent of the operating costs. States must set safety standards that are at least as effective as the comparable federal standards. Typically, state-level programs adopt standards that are identical to OSHA, although states have the option to establish standards not addressed by federal rules.

OSHA has also created local emphasis programs (LEPs) – enforcement strategies designed and implemented by OSHA regional or area offices. LEPs address hazards that pose a risk to employees in the given jurisdiction. They typically include increasing awareness of specific hazards and programs to reduce or eliminate them. The group practice administrator should be aware of local LEPs that focus on standards applicable to the practice.

The creation of an effective OSHA compliance program is a substantial responsibility for the medical practice administrator. The complexity and diversity of OSHA standards are significant, and developing an effective program requires more than a cut-and-paste approach. Keys to success are organizational buy-in at all levels, employee involvement in identifying potential workplace hazards and solutions, training and documentation, and constant review of the work environment and evolving OSHA standards.

OSHA e-Tools

OSHA has developed a series of standalone, interactive, Web-based training tools on safety and health topics. They provide information and advice on how OSHA standards apply to a work site. The medical practice administrator will find the following tools invaluable in understanding the applicability of OSHA regulations to the development of an OSHA compliance plan:

- Hospital e-tool – www.osha.gov/SLTC/etools/hospital/main-page.html
- Evacuation Plans and Procedures e-tool – www.osha.gov/SLTC/etools/evacuation/index.html

OSHA Website Resources

OSHA Notice of Employee Rights – Available as a print-ready pdf file in English (www.osha.gov/Publications/osha3165.pdf) or Spanish (www.osha.gov/Publications/osha3167.pdf).

Record-keeping forms – Available at www.osha.gov/recordkeeping/Rkforms.html. Form 300, Log of Work-Related Injuries and Illnesses; Form 301, Injuries and Illness Incident Report; and Form 300A, Summary of Work-Related Injuries and Illnesses may be downloaded as pdf files or Microsoft® *Excel* spreadsheets.

The OSHA handbook of all record-keeping requirements is available at www.osha.gov/Publications/recordkeeping/OSHA_3245_REVISED.pdf.

Small Business Handbook – An excellent overview of OSHA requirements and resources. Available as either a pdf file (www.osha.gov/Publications/smallbusiness/small-business.pdf) or an html file (www.osha.gov/Publications/smallbusiness/small-business.html).

Personnel protective equipment – This overview is available as either a pdf file (www.osha.gov/Publications/osha3151.pdf) or an html file (www.osha.gov/Publications/osha3151.html).

Bloodborne pathogens and hazard communications – This handbook combines these two standards in either a pdf file (www.osha.gov/Publications/osha3186.pdf) or an html file (www.osha.gov/Publications/osha3186.html).

Needlestick safety programs – "Safer Medical Device Implementation in Health Care Facilities: Sharing Lessons Learned" is available on the NIOSH Website (www.cdc.gov/niosh/topics/bbp/safer/).

"Workbook for Designing, Implementing, and Evaluating a Sharps Injury Prevention Program" is available on the Centers for Disease Control and Prevention Website: (www.cdc.gov/sharpssafety/).

Record-Keeping

Similar to patient records and other business records, records of government contracts and all aspects of the corporate compliance program should be maintained in accordance with contract specifications and with the federal regulations relevant to each specific federal act.

Complying with the Law[52]

Practice administrators and physicians alike should be aware of several legal issues applicable to any business, including medical practices. Not intended as an in-depth analysis, this brief overview spotlights relevant legal principles regarding the organization and operation of a group practice. This includes issues related to antitrust, fraud and abuse, and other legal or regulatory concerns. Legal issues related to credentialing and legal structure are covered in books related to organizational governance.

Antitrust Laws

Many federal and state laws affect medical practices. A prime example is antitrust regulations. There are numerous federal antitrust laws, including the Sherman Act, the Clayton Act, and the Federal Trade Commission Act, as well as similar state laws. Practice administrators won't need to memorize the specifics of these laws, but they should understand the basic requirements and what they prohibit.

As a general matter, antitrust laws are designed to promote and protect competition – to eliminate restraints of trade and related activities that interfere with competition. They are based on the theory that a competitive marketplace will be good for consumers by resulting in lower prices for goods and services and the development of new products. Accordingly, all antitrust laws are generally designed to promote and protect competition, and to prevent actions viewed to be contrary to a well-functioning, competitive marketplace.

All antitrust laws are complex, and their application to a particular circumstance will always depend on the particular facts and situation at hand. Nonetheless, given their focus on competition, two of the broad areas that antitrust laws focus on relate to:

- The size and power of organizations in a particular marketplace – commonly referred to as concerns with market power or the creation of a prohibited "monopoly"; and

- Prohibited "joint action" where organizations or individuals that would otherwise be competing with each other, collude or jointly engage in other anticompetitive conduct. These laws prohibit any agreement between two or more competitors to restrain trade, such as price fixing; refusing to deal with certain third parties; and agreeing to allocate or divide markets.

In particular, it is important to understand that:

- Practices cannot combine or merge for the sole purpose of creating a monopoly (i.e., a medical practice that is so large and powerful that it can set prices and otherwise restrict competition); and

- Physicians and practices who are otherwise competitors cannot confer with or engage in prohibited "joint action" with other physicians or practices for the purpose of setting fees or refusing to deal with third parties, such as insurers and hospitals; and

- Practices cannot reach agreements regarding the allocation or division of markets (e.g., one practice agrees with another practice that each will only provide services at a particular hospital, in a particular part of town or to only certain third-party payers).

Medical practices must keep these antitrust restrictions in mind when considering entering into joint ventures and negotiating payer contracts. Federal antitrust prohibitions are summarized in Exhibit 1.

Federal antitrust laws may be enforced by federal officials, by state attorneys general, and through private lawsuits brought by individuals or organizations claiming to have suffered injury to their

---

EXHIBIT 1

Summary of Federal Antitrust Prohibitions

- Sherman Antitrust Act, Section 1: Prohibits contracts, combinations, and conspiracies that unreasonably restrain trade.

- Sherman Antitrust Act, Section 2: Prohibits monopolization, attempted monopolization, or combinations and conspiracies to monopolize.

- Clayton Antitrust Act, Section 7: Prohibits mergers, acquisitions, and certain joint ventures where the likely effect may be to substantially lessen competition or tend to create a monopoly.

- Federal Trade Commission Act, Section 5: Prohibits unfair methods of competition, including unfair advertising and unfair or deceptive business practices.

- Robinson-Patman Act, Section 3: Prohibits price discrimination in the sale of certain commodities.

businesses or property due to alleged anticompetitive conduct. State antitrust laws may generally be enforced by a state's attorney general and private-party suits. Potential private parties include other individual and organizational competitors in the health care delivery market who may claim to have been injured by allegedly anticompetitive conduct.

Fraud and Abuse Prohibitions

Experienced practice administrators have likely encountered a heavy emphasis on health care fraud and abuse prevention in their careers. Medicare and Medicaid laws impose a variety of restrictions designed to prohibit fraud and abuse that impacts these programs. Some prohibitions deal with activities such as submitting false claims for reimbursement, making false representations, and other misrepresentations-of-fact activities. A second set of prohibitions addresses activities considered abuse of the Medicare or Medicaid programs – the antikickback prohibitions and the interrelated Ethics in Patient Referrals Act, also known as the Stark law (named for the act's sponsor, U.S. Representative Pete Stark.)

Stark Laws

Stark law refers to physician self-referral. Stark I (Omnibus Budget Reconciliation Act of 1989) restricts or prohibits referring Medicare or Medicaid patients to clinical laboratory services in which the referring physician (or an immediate family member) has a financial or ownership interest. Stark II (Omnibus Budget Reconciliation Act of 1993) added further restrictions for additional designated health services and provided exemptions when these services are provided by physician group practices.

Stark III (i.e., "Phase III") made multiple changes and clarified many previous issues, and it became effective Dec. 4, 2007. While it is mandatory to obtain expert legal advice – this chapter in no way provides the extensive navigation required through the maze of Stark laws and other antikickback statutes – it is imperative that all providers in all settings of practice have appropriate knowledge of the Stark laws (and its exceptions), the antikickback statute, and safe harbors. Penalties for violating Stark laws are severe, including fines of up to $15,000 per service and the economic threat of exclusion from participation in federal health care programs, which may result in exclusion of any type of health care program and loss of privileges at hospitals and surgery centers.

The additional designated health services include:

- Physical therapy services;

- Occupational therapy services;

- Radiology services (including magnetic resonance imaging, computerized axial tomography, and ultrasound);

- Radiation therapy services and supplies;

- Durable medical equipment and supplies;

- Prosthetics, orthotics, and prosthetic devices and supplies;

- Home health services;

- Outpatient prescription drugs; and

- Inpatient and outpatient hospital services.

These Stark regulations also stipulate how physicians may receive compensation related to providing these designated health services. Physicians can receive compensation based directly on the services that the physician personally performs, but not on the technical component.

Antikickback Law Summary

The antikickback law was enacted by Congress to eliminate Medicare and Medicaid abuses that increase program costs. In brief, federal and state laws prohibit the payment of any remuneration for health care–related referrals. The antikickback prohibition provides for the imposition of criminal penalties (a $25,000 fine, imprisonment up to five years, or both) upon anyone who knowingly and willfully offers, pays, solicits, or receives any remuneration (anything of value) directly, indirectly, overtly, or covertly, in cash or in kind, in return for referring an individual to a person for the furnishing or arranging for services for which payment may be made by Medicare or Medicaid. The prohibitions also cover recommending the purchase, lease, order, or arrangement for any good, facility, service, or item for which payment may be made under the Medicare or Medicaid programs.

The Department of Health and Human Services (HHS) Office of Inspector General (OIG) periodically publishes "fraud alerts" that describe business practices and arrangements that could be in violation of the law. Fraud alerts can be used to illustrate questionable practices that might run afoul of the antikickback law. These have included:

- Prescription drug marketing schemes;

- Clinical laboratory activities such as lab-pricing arrangements, provision of phlebotomy services to physicians, and other arrangements;

- Joint-venture arrangements between those in a position to refer business such as physicians and those providing items and services such as medical equipment suppliers, laboratory services, and others;

- Routine waiver of copayments or deductibles under Medicare Part B by providers paid on a reasonable charge basis;

- Hospital incentives to physicians; and

- Provision of medical supplies to nursing facilities.

State laws also impose similar requirements and restrictions; for example, prohibitions on fee splitting. In both federal and state situations, legal counsel with expertise in interpreting these ever-evolving laws is necessary.

CMS is responsible for ensuring proper billing and reimbursement for health services provided to Medicare and Medicaid enrollees.

In Medicare, the most common forms of fraud include:

- Billing for services not furnished;

- Misrepresenting the diagnosis to justify payment;

- Soliciting, offering, or receiving a kickback;

- Unbundling or "exploding" charges;

- Falsifying certificates of medical necessity, plans of treatment, and medical records to justify payment; and

- Billing for a service not furnished as billed (i.e., upcoding).

CMS and the HHS OIG will also prosecute practices for routinely waiving copayments.

It is up to each physician and medical practice to follow proper coding and billing procedures to ensure compliance with Medicare regulations. Many private insurers have similar fraud and abuse policies and audits in place, so it is advisable to remain vigilant with all patient practices, Medicare and non-Medicare alike.

Other Legal and/or Regulatory Concerns

Practice administrators must be sure to recognize additional legal and/or regulatory issues that may arise in connection with business activities. These include:

- *Anti-discrimination provisions* including the federal civil rights acts, the Americans with Disabilities Act, and analogous state law provisions. Such laws typically affect an organization's employment practices, as well as the way in which the enterprise conducts business. Other health care–specific laws are also in effect, such as the federal Emergency Medical Treatment and Active Labor Act and analogous state laws related to "patient dumping" provisions.

- *Certificate of Need laws* that may arise in connection with the creation of new provider capabilities (e.g., the establishment of outpatient surgical centers, community clinics, or other enterprises), or in connection with changes in a provider's business structure and business capabilities (e.g., the number of licensed beds in a hospital). Such laws are typically found in state statutes and their implementing regulations.

- *Clinical Laboratory Improvement Act* and other federal and state licensing and/or certification statutes that affect the operational aspects of health care delivery. CMS regulates all laboratory testing (except research) performed on humans in the United States through Clinical Laboratory Improvement Amendments (CLIA). The objective of the CLIA program is to ensure quality laboratory testing. Leaders of a medical organization must decide the level of certification it will apply for. Many practices simply apply for a certificate of waiver, which allows the office laboratory to perform only very simple tests such as a stick glucose test. However, if there is any physician-performed microscopy, the practice must apply for full certification.

- *Confidentiality and medical records laws,* such as HIPAA, that have significant implications for record retention, medical record confidentiality, access to records, copying costs, and many other issues involving the delivery of health care and the conduct of business activities.

- *Contract law* governing the terms of various contractual arrangements.

- *Employment-related laws*, including federal provisions governing ways and other terms of employment such as the Fair Labor Standards Act, workplace safety concerns such as the Occupational Safety and Health Act, requirements of state workers' compensation laws, and other state law provisions governing payment of wages, working conditions, and additional employment factors.

- *Environmental laws* based in federal and state statutes that define requirements related to the production and disposal of waste and that impose liability for cleanup of hazardous materials and related provisions.

- *Facilities licensure provisions* that require separate licenses for different types of health care–related transactions, including the development of ancillary services, outpatient clinics, and others.

- *Health Care Quality Improvement Act* and other laws related to provider credentialing activities. Certain statutes provide limited immunity for peer review activities as well as traditional medical staff activities. Provider organizations may have an obligation to provide reports to, and obtain periodic information from, the National Practitioner Data Bank in connection with their credentialing and peer-review activities.

- *Health Insurance Portability and Accountability Act of 1996 (HIPAA)* that covers three major areas: ensuring portable health coverage for workers when they lose their jobs or change employers, reducing fraud and abuse in the health care system, and standardizing the electronic transmission of health data. The act requires health care entities to set up systems for secure electronic transactions. This act also triggered regulations governing the confidentiality of all types of medical information. Health care entities are required to designate a privacy official, provide privacy training to employees, implement safeguards to protect health information from intentional or accidental misuse, provide a means for individuals to file complaints about the entity's information practices, and develop a system of sanctions for employees and business partners who violate the entity's policies. HIPAA encompasses medical group practice operations, especially registration, medical records and telephone, fax and Internet usage. Noncompliance carries heavy penalties.

Included in HIPAA is the administrative simplification section with an intent to simplify the administrative burden faced by the health care industry. Lawmakers sought to standardize the electronic transmission of health data and facilitate transition from paper to electronic claims. The law required the HHS secretary to adopt national standards for identifiers, transactions, claims attachment, health data privacy and security, and medical records.

Health care providers who choose to transmit claims electronically must comply with the standards, though they may contract with clearinghouses to conduct standard transactions for them.

It is critical that medical practices comply with the HIPAA privacy regulations. Medical practices must protect the confidentiality and privacy of patient information in any format (spoken, print, or electronic). Practices must also provide individuals with access to their health information following the provisions of the act. More information is available at the CMS Website, http://www.cms.hhs.gov/.

- *Payment reimbursement provisions* including those of the federal Medicare law governing provider reimbursement, provider numbers, the appropriate method of billing, and other concerns.

- *Professional negligence/malpractice* including new liability concerns raised in the context of managed care. Such issues can arise in connection with an individual provider's response to utilization review determinations, the activities of provider organizations in undertaking utilization review, credentialing, and other activities. Provider organizations may require their own separate policies of medical malpractice and general liability insurance.

- *Public institution/pubic finance issues* that may arise in connection with business activities undertaken by public institutions such as county or district hospitals, academic medical centers and similar public and/or quasi-public organizations. Restrictions on the types of business arrangements and activities that may be undertaken by such enterprises, their use of public funds, and other requirements may be imposed through a variety of different means, including state constitutions, statutes, bond covenants, and others.

- *Tax laws* that affect both the form of business enterprises and the manner of their operation. In some states, certain types of organizations (e.g., professional service corporations) are subject to excise taxes, gross receipts taxes, and similar tax obligations, whereas other enterprises (e.g., limited liability companies) are not. A wide variety of sales, use, and other taxes may be imposed on health care–related enterprises and their business activities. Moreover, federal, state, and local tax laws each has its own reporting, payment, and other operational requirements that must be followed.

- *Zoning and land use restrictions* that may affect the types of activities undertaken at different locations in a community. Such provisions may affect the business options available to physicians, hospitals, and other providers including the development of outpatient service centers, joint venture arrangements, and similar enterprises.

Corporate Compliance

The government recently began encouraging corporate compliance programs for all health care organizations. It does not *require* medical group practices to implement such programs; however, it actively encourages voluntary compliance efforts and self-policing, and it has a strong enforcement effort, particularly related to Medicare and Medicaid fraud and abuse. Whether a health care billing entity has a corporate compliance program in place may determine whether a violation of a federal requirement is treated as an innocent mistake or as a fraudulent act.

Because it is not required, some practices may not have a compliance program or officer. Putting one in place depends on the size of the group, the complexity of its operations and regulatory responsibilities, and its ability to develop and implement a plan – and to live by it.

A corporate compliance plan states the group's intention to prevent criminal acts by employees, to encourage ethical conduct, and to reduce the impact of any sanctions that may be imposed. The compliance plan says the practice will:

- Establish, maintain, and revise as necessary compliance standards and procedures to be followed by its employees and other agents that are reasonably capable of reducing the prospect of criminal conduct;

- Assign a senior manager (a compliance "officer") the overall responsibility to oversee compliance with such standards and procedures and to report noncompliance to the board of directors;

- Use due care not to delegate substantial discretionary authority to individuals whom the organization knows, through the exercise of due diligence, have a propensity to engage in illegal activities by conducting licensure and criminal background checks;

- Communicate its compliance standards and procedures to all employees and other agents via the employee handbook, a code of conduct, and ongoing training;

- Take reasonable steps, such as audits and monitoring systems, to achieve compliance;

- Enforce these mechanisms through appropriate disciplinary avenues; and

- Respond appropriately to any offense and seek to prevent similar offenses including any necessary modifications to the program to prevent and detect violations of law.

Knowing that the government imposes heavy penalties on non-compliance, especially related to fraud and abuse, it behooves a group practice to develop and implement a corporate compliance program.

Conclusion

RISK MANAGEMENT is a comprehensive set of management skills that covers the entire spectrum of activity in the practice. It is not a function; rather, it is a management skill and process that, if used correctly, can identify areas of potential loss long before they emerge. Risk management draws on federal and state legislation and regulation as well as principles of safety science, principles of communication and human interaction, and business practices. It creates a network of measurements against which the daily operation of the medical practice can benchmark itself to find the means to reduce injury to patients and employees and to minimize financial loss to the health care organization.

Exercises

THESE QUESTIONS have been retired from the ACMPE Essay Exam question bank. Because there are so many ways to handle various situations, there are no "right" answers, and thus, no answer key. Use these questions to help you practice responses in different scenarios.

1. You are the new administrator of a specialty group practice with a 50-percent Medicare patient population. You are made aware that one physician in particular has not dictated consultation reports back to the referring physicians for up to one year. The practice has, however, billed and been paid for these consultations. You are concerned about the compliance issues surrounding this problem.

   Describe how you would handle this situation.

2. You are the administrator of a small medical practice. You and the physicians recently attended a meeting at which Medicare fraud and abuse was a hot topic. The physicians are now convinced that a compliance program is needed in their practice and have asked you to develop one.

Describe how you would develop, implement, and monitor the compliance program.

3. You are the administrator of a medical group. A patient has contacted you, claiming that his outstanding bill is the result of incorrect billing practices, and the billing office is unwilling to correct the invoice. The patient has contacted his attorney about filing a complaint with the Board of Medical Examiners, as well as filing a consumer fraud claim.

   Describe how you would handle this situation.

4. You are the administrator for a 10-physician group prac-
    tice. Two weeks ago, a physician's nurse resigned to
    accept a position at another clinic. Today you received,
    by registered mail, a notice from the Equal Employment
    Opportunity Commission stating that the former employee
    has filed a charge of discrimination against the practice.
    She alleges that she was sexually harassed by the physician
    with whom she worked.

    Explain how you would handle this situation.

5. You are the administrator of a large multispecialty group. At the last board of director's monthly meeting, your group adopted a compliance plan proposed by the compliance committee. The compliance committee is made up of five senior members who volunteered for the committee. A number of physicians are noncompliant with the plan. The pediatricians in the group feel there is no need for them to meet the plan guidelines because they do not treat Medicare patients. The two rheumatologists in the group, who are not compliance committee members, do not feel they have to meet the plan guidelines either. Two cardiologists who serve on the compliance committee want to know if they will get extra compensation if they meet the compliance plan guidelines.

   Describe how you would handle this situation.

6. You are the administrator of a midsize primary care practice that recently had to eliminate several positions because of declining reimbursements. You receive an anonymous response to an exit interview questionnaire from a former employee. The document states that the employee had concerns about inappropriate behavior in the practice. The employee shared that one of the doctors routinely upcoded, that all employees and physicians were aware of the situation, and that no one responded to concerns about this wrongdoing. You bring this complaint to the compliance officer, who is concerned that the former employee may become a whistleblower.

Describe how you would handle this situation.

Notes

1. G. L. Head and S. Horn, *Essentials of Risk Management,* Vol. 1 (Malvern, PA: Insurance Institute of America, 1991), 1.

2. J. McCaffrey and S. Hagg-Rickert, "Development of a Risk Management Program," in *The Risk Management Handbook for Healthcare Organizations*, ed. R. Carroll (San Francisco: Jossey-Bass, 2004), 95.

3. W. R. Ching, "Enterprise Risk Management: Laying a Broader Framework for Health Care Risk Management," in *The Risk Management Handbook for Healthcare Organizations*, ed. R. Carroll (San Francisco: Jossey-Bass, 2004), 3.

4. Head and Horn, *Essentials*, Vol. 1, 6.

5. J. Reason, *Human Error* (Cambridge, UK: Cambridge University Press, 1990), 208.

6. K. B. Thomas, "New Orleans Today: It's Worse Than You Think," *Time* (November 20, 2005).

7. Reason, *Human Error*, 208.

8. R. E. McDermott, R. J. Mikulak, and M. R. Beauregard, *The Basics of FMEA* (Portland, OR: Productivity, 1996), 1–5.

9. Head and Horn, *Essentials*, Vol. 1, 8.

10. G. L. Head and S. Horn, *Essentials of Risk Management*, Vol. 2 (Malvern, PA: Insurance Institute of America, 1991), 13.

11. For more information, see the "Patient and Provider Education Materials" section on the Centers for Disease Control Website, www.cdc.gov/flu/professionals/patiented.htm.

12. For information on infection control recommendations for pandemic influenza, see "Supplement 4 Infection Control" on the HHS Website, www.hhs.gov/pandemicflu/plan/sup4.html.

13. For more information, see "Surge Capacity" in "Supplement 3 Healthcare Planning" on the HHS Website, www.hhs.gov/pandemicflu/plan/sup3.html#surge.

14. House Committee on Science, World Trade Center, "Lessons Learned from Ground Zero," www.house.gov/science/wtc.htm (accessed March 7, 2002).

15. K. R. Roberts, K. Yu, and D. V. Stralen, "Patient Safety Is an Organizational Systems Issue: Lessons from a Variety of Industries," in *The Patient Safety Handbook*, eds. B. Youngberg and M. Hatlie (Sudbury, MA: Jones and Bartlett, 2004), 171–173.

16. Ibid.

17. G. Porto, "Creating Patient Safety and High Reliability," in *The Risk Management Handbook for Healthcare Organizations*, ed. R. Carroll (San Francisco: Jossey-Bass, 2004), 322.

18. Head and Horn, *Essentials*, Vol. 2, 40.

19. Ibid., 162.

20. American College of Medical Practice Executives (ACMPE), *The ACMPE Guide to the Body of Knowledge for Medical Practice Management* (Englewood, CO: ACMPE, 2003), 76.

21. A portion of this chapter is reprinted from *HR Policies and Procedures Manual for Medical Practices*, 4th edition, copyright 2007, pages 225–233, with permission of Medical Group Management Association. All rights reserved.

22. Drug Free Workplace Act of 1988, U.S. Code 41, §701.

23. P. J. White, "Employment Practices Legal Issues," 873.

24. P. D. Stergios, et al., "Labor and Employment Laws Applicable to Physicians' Practices," in *Physician Practice Management*, ed. L. F. Wolper (Sudbury, MA: Jones and Bartlett, 2005), 536-538.

25. Fair Labor Standards Act, U.S. Code 29, Ch. 8, §201 et seq.

26. Equal Pay Act of 1963, U.S. Code 29, §206(d)(1) et seq.

27. Title VII of the Civil Rights Act of 1964, 29 CFR Part 1604.11.

28. Americans with Disabilities Act of 1990, U.S. Code 42, §12101 et seq.

29. Drug Abuse Prevention, Treatment, and Rehabilitation Act, 42 CFR Part 2.

30. P. A. Nakamura, "Contract Review Primer for Risk Managers," in *The Risk Management Handbook for Healthcare Organizations*, ed. R. Carroll (San Francisco: Jossey-Bass, 2004), 500.

31. Ibid., 489–491.

32. J. McCaffrey and S. Hagg-Rickert, "Development of a Risk Management Program," 104.

33. J. Horty and M. Hanslovan, "Governance of the Health Care Organization," in *The Risk Management Handbook for Healthcare Organizations*, ed. R. Carroll (San Francisco: Jossey-Bass, 2004), 83.

34. Safe Medical Device Act of 1990, U.S. Code 21 §360i(a).

35. Ibid., 360i(a)(6).

36. This chapter was written by Lorraine C. Woods, FACMPE, and is reprinted with permission from MGMA, as derived from a professional paper submitted to the American College of Medical Practice Executives in partial fulfillment of requirements to achieve the certification of Fellow.

37. Andrew Hiles, *Business Continuity: Best Practices*, 2nd ed. (Brookfield: Rothstein Associates, 2004), 3.

38. Aktar Syed and Afsar Syed, *Business Continuity Planning and Methodology* (Canada: SentryX, 2004), 1.

39. Jay Moore, "Patching New Orleans," *HealthLeaders* (August 2006): 21.

40. Hiles, 41.

41. Syed and Syed, 9.

42. Gary Bennett, "Managing Risk for Clients and for Ourselves. A Bug's Life (and the Turnbull Report)," *Risk Management at PB: Balancing Risk and Reward XVI*, no. 51 (January 2002), 3.

43. Hiles, 29.

44. Syed and Syed, 108.

45. Hiles, 208.

46. Hiles, 26.

47. Michael Wallace and Lawrence Webber, *The Disaster Recovery Handbook* (New York: AMACOM, 2004) 127.

48. Wallace, 206.

49. Government Policy Newslinks, available at http://policynewslinks.com.

50. This section was adapted from an article in *MGMA Connexion* (August 2007), which was a professional paper submitted to the American College of Medical Practice Executives in partial fulfillment of requirements to achieve the certification of Fellow. Reprinted with permission of the Medical Group Management Association.

51. Occupational Safety and Health Administration (2005). *Small Business Handbook* (2209-02R): 10–13.

52. The "Complying with the Law" section is reprinted with permission from the Medical Group Management Association. It appears on pages 15–26 of *Rx for Business Success: Joining a Medical Practice*, copyright 2005.

Bibliography

Bennett, Gary. "Managing Risk for Clients and for Ourselves. A Bug's Life (and the Turnbull Report)." *Risk Management at PB: Balancing Risk and Reward* XVI, no. 51 (January 2002), www.pbworld.com (accessed Dec. 12, 2006).

"Blackout Survival Guide." *Popular Mechanics* (July 21, 2006), www.popularmechanics.com (accessed July 27, 2006).

Gurchiek, Kathy. "Ruth's Chris Provides a Lesson in Disaster Planning." *SHRM* (January 5, 2006), www.shrm.org/hrnews (accessed Jan. 10, 2006).

Hagland, Mark. "Disaster Response: The Many Heroes of Katrina." *Healthcare Informatics* (November 2005): 10–16.

Hiles, Andrew. *Business Continuity: Best Practices*, 2nd ed. Brookfield: Rothstein Associates, 2004.

Kramer, Stacey. "Prepping for Disaster." *Healthcare Informatics* (August 2006): 62.

Moore, Jay. "Patching New Orleans." *HealthLeaders* (August 2006): 20–27.

Reynolds, Glenn. "When Your City Goes Dark, Preparing for Power Failure." *MSNBC* July 25, 2006), www.glennreynolds.com (accessed July 27, 2006).

Simms, Frederick R. Jr. "Stormy Weather, Preparing for and Recovering From Disasters." *MGMA Connexion* (January 2006): 44–47.

Syed, Aktar, and Afsar Syed. *Business Continuity Planning and Methodology*. Canada: SentryX, 2004.

Wallace, Michael, and Lawrence Webber. *The Disaster Recovery Handbook*. New York: AMACOM, 2004.

Woodward, Nancy Hatch. "Pandemic, How to Prepare for the Unthinkable." *HR Magazine* (May 2006): 46–52.

Index

Note: (ex.) indicates exhibit.